SAVED BY THE MOUTH

Saved by the
MOUTH

Be Healthier, Save Money, and
Live Longer by Improving Your Oral Health

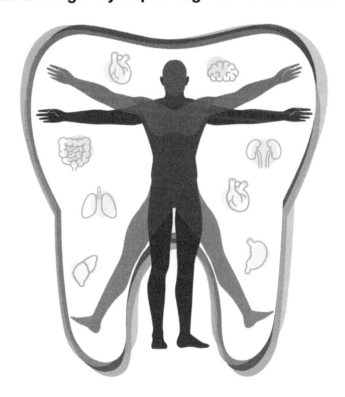

Katie Lee, DDS

LIONCREST
PUBLISHING

SAVED BY THE MOUTH
Be Healthier, Save Money, and Live Longer
by Improving Your Oral Health

FIRST EDITION

ISBN		
978-1-5445-4025-2	*Hardcover*	
978-1-5445-4026-9	*Paperback*	
978-1-5445-4027-6	*Ebook*	
978-1-5445-4028-3	*Audiobook*	

I dedicate this book to my husband, Doug, whose unconditional love and support give me the courage to do hard things.

Contents

Foreword

—DR. VICTORIA SAMPSON

I AM HONOURED TO BE ASKED TO WRITE THIS FOREWORD, not only because Katie Lee has been an inspirational visionary in the world of dentistry, but also because I passionately believe in the value this book brings.

I met Katie in 2022 when we were both speaking at a conference. I was asked to cancel my afternoon of patients and fly in one night earlier to have dinner with a 'woman I would love and be inspired by' before the conference started. The invitation was too good to pass up, and there I was, on my way to dinner in Frankfurt the next day. Katie exceeded my expectations, and we spent the rest of that evening talking about microbiome testing and salivary diagnostics, and sharing tips on how we can treat patients holistically (what better dinner table conversation?!). For years I was seen as an 'out of the box thinker'. Many would question why I thought the mouth was connected to the rest of the body or why I would 'waste time on microbiome testing when [I] could make triple by slapping on some veneers'.

I had never met a dentist like Katie, who shared the same views as I did yet somehow was able to strike a beautiful balance between being caring, successful, and innovative.

After decades of dentistry and medicine being separate entities, Katie is spearheading the movement reconnecting the two together to enable full-body health of our patients. In 490 BC, Hippocrates, the 'father of medicine', strongly believed in the importance the mouth had in whole-body health. He even remarked he cured rheumatoid arthritis once by removing an infected tooth. Unfortunately, when medical schools first opened in 1765, the mouth was not included in the syllabus, resulting in a separate school of dentistry forming in 1840. Since then, doctors and dentists have traditionally worked separately, rarely joining forces. Fast-forward centuries and we are now understanding that the body is a delicate interplay between numerous systems. When one system is down, for example, the liver, this can have implications elsewhere in the body. If we truly want optimal full-body health, we must consider every system in the body. One question that crops up is 'But how are these systems all connected?'

In 2009 when the Human Microbiome Project was founded, we started to understand the importance of not only the gut microbiome, but also the oral microbiome. We realised that we have numerous microbiomes that all work together and are also directly impacted by our habits and lifestyles.

Reading this book, you will find it hard to not see how the mouth is connected to the rest of the body and what impact a healthy mouth can have elsewhere. If this book doesn't convince you to pick up your toothbrush, I don't know what will.

Introduction

"She looked as beautiful as if she had been dead."

—*PHANTOM OF THE OPERA*

I TIPPED MY HEAD AWAY FROM THE WIND, TURNING IT back for just a second, so I could hear my girlfriend better. She sat behind me on my ATV, yelling something in my ear as we raced down the road.

We'd just come back from spending the first part of the day at the lake, laughing and talking and daydreaming with the optimism of young girls who hadn't had their hearts broken or been stung by the realities of adult life. But the bees were buzzing.

There was a bump, a jolt, and then blackness.

Much later, according to my parents, I walked a half mile down the road, made it to someone's house, knocked on their door, and asked for my friend and me to be taken to the hospital before I collapsed. That's what a body in shock can do. I don't remember any of that. I do remember hearing voices, though I couldn't really see. I heard my mother sobbing, my father consoling her, and the doctors frantically trying to keep both of them calm. Apparently, I went headfirst—while not wearing a helmet—into a telephone pole at over thirty miles per hour. I'd broken my face—literally. Every bone in my face from the eyebrows down was broken. I was missing part of my lip and a few teeth (they were stuck in the telephone pole).

I briefly wake up later that day to monsters in masks and scrubs, to bright lights above me, and to pain so intense that my body wants me to go unconscious again. I know I'm going to die. I'm convinced of it. I close my eyes and try to get it over with. I just hope I didn't kill my friend too.

Several days later, I wake up alone in a hospital room, nauseous and with the kind of sweats you get right before you throw up. Reflexively, I try to take a deep breath, only to discover my mouth won't open. It's wired shut. I panic. Jolted, I try to touch my face and watch, in horror, as my bloodied, swollen knuckles extending from a casted arm near my face. I am able to twist my arm enough for my fingertips to touch what feels like something that isn't part of my body. The surface of my face is so foreign, it might as well be the moon: sandy in spots, covered in rough stitches in others. There is no feeling on the right side or on my lips. The only way I know I'm touching them is because I can feel my trembling fingers run across the bridge of my broken nose.

I'm alive, but barely. I've been in a coma for nearly a week and have lost over ten pounds, which is catastrophic for a broken body fighting hard to survive. My parents have been promised so many times that I am going to die, be a vegetable, or never be the same again after the damage from my head heals that they've started to make arrangements for any of those outcomes.

But I'm a fighter. Somewhere, somehow, between the surgeries and the haze of painkillers, I manage to put on my gloves.

Long story short: that's how I got into dentistry.

MEET DR. KATIE LEE (FORMERLY KNOWN AS FUCK FACE)

No one knew how to tell me what happened. I heard them talking about strategies on how to explain my situation to me. But I already knew I was mangled. I saw my face when I was rolled down for some X-rays. They were the kind of X-rays where there's a mirror in front of you because you have to line up your nose with the lasers. It was the first time I realized I looked like a scary alien. But I could only see what had happened on the outside. Inside my body, things weren't any better—particularly in my mouth.

My mouth had been wired shut so my jaws could heal. If you've never had your mouth wired shut, let me assure you it's as bad as it sounds. And it wasn't just wires. There were plates, screws, nuts, and bolts holding my face together. That meant there was no eating anything that needed to be chewed and there was no brushing of the teeth. And when the pain meds made me vomit, well…you get the picture. My broken teeth that were left in my mouth just rotted in the mire. On top of that, my parents, who only wanted me to experience whatever joy I could in life, for the next eight weeks fed me things like ice cream with chocolate sauce and liquidy mashed potatoes through a straw. You know, things that aren't the best choice to sit for hours/days on your teeth.

Compounding it all was the weight loss: I was malnourished, severely. To the point that my internal organs had begun to shut down. Body processes that weren't necessary for life were put on hold by my system just to maintain survival. So things like teeth remineralizing didn't happen.

But guess what did happen? Two months later, school started

as usual that fall. I began my freshman year looking and feeling like a freak of nature—a freak of nature with missing front teeth. Teenagers, in their cruel lack of wisdom and compassion, had great fun with me. Fuck Face became my name.

But I got the last laugh. The fighter who flexed her muscles while in a coma managed to make one hell of a comeback. Similarly to how God took one of Adam's ribs and used it to make Eve, my doctors (nine surgeries later) used one of mine to reconstruct my jaw and save my face.

I had a surgery about every six months. I'd study as hard as I could so I could take my exams early, and then have surgery. Rinse and repeat until I had my final surgery my senior year and was able to open my mouth and get teeth implants.

To say high school was tough is an understatement. Medical issues aside, psychologically and emotionally I took a beating. The taunting, teasing, and bullying just ate at me. But it also made me determined to prove something to those kids. I put my head down and just focused on doing my best at whatever I was doing. I became the captain of every sport I was in and wound up becoming the valedictorian of my class. (Take *that*, assholes.)

And I became determined to be the best dentist I could be. See, while my face and jaws healed during high school, I had holes in my smile. The trauma that did to my psyche was so profound…I don't want anyone to take any kind of hit to their self-esteem because of their teeth. It turned me into a self-conscious introvert who avoided smiling and social interactions.

But as I grew in my profession, I realized that a good, healthy smile means more than just having a pretty face or feeling confident walking down a high school hallway. It means you have a healthy body too. So my main focus throughout my career has been to remain at the cutting edge of dental care.

I have been able to partner with dentists all over the country and train them on how to improve their patients' oral and systemic health. I decided to write this book so that the patients themselves would be informed as well. By hitting from both sides, dentists and patients, my hope is that we will have a much healthier population where everyone can thrive.

In your hands is proof that your oral health is the key to your overall health, wellness, and longevity. Learn from it. Then discuss with your dentist what you can do as a team to address what's going on in your mouth that could be impacting your whole body and your wallet.

THE MOUTH-BODY-BANK ACCOUNT CONNECTION

I'll begin in Part 1 with a general overview of the odds of being healthy in the United States and what's making it so difficult for us to maintain our health in general (hint: inflammation!). You'll learn how inflammation works to create disease and/or makes diseases worse. You'll see how the mouth is often where the problems start, even when they manifest their worst symptoms elsewhere in the body.

In Part 2, I discuss the specifics of different diseases and how they are impacted by your oral health. You'll discover that by examining and treating what's going on in the mouth, we can often find the beginnings of causal pathways that lead to conditions like heart disease, diabetes, cancer, inflammatory conditions such as irritable bowel syndrome and rheumatoid arthritis, sleep apnea, reproduction and fertility problems, and even Alzheimer's and dementia. Even better: by treating those issues in the mouth, we can improve the health of those patients and help manage or even cure them.

Because the point of this book is to offer hope, prevention, and solutions, Part 3 goes into what you and your dentist can do to improve your oral health, which means improving the health of your whole body, which is what will save you big bucks in the long haul. Chapters 10 and 11 will cover what you can do for yourself, and Chapters 12 and 13 will discuss what you can talk to your dentist about.

I'll end the book with a template for you to create your own Personal Wellness Plan and encourage you to make a commitment to maintaining the best oral care you can. I truly do want you to have not just a gorgeous smile, but a healthy and gorgeous smile. As my opening story proves, I know firsthand the importance of that.

I also know firsthand how intimidating it can be to go to the dentist. Spending time with us is usually not on any top-ten lists of fun things to do. And I get it. Dentists haven't always been the compassionate and educated professionals we are today. But the profession has changed tremendously over the past couple of decades, and even more so since it began. We no longer have barbers offering to pull your tooth at the end of your haircut (I kid you not).

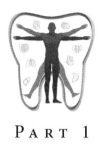

PART 1

THE STATE OF HEALTH
IN THE UNION

CHAPTER 1

Health in the USA

DEBRAH HAD BEEN A PATIENT OF MINE FOR THE LAST eight years of my active practice. Like clockwork, she showed up every six months as if her life depended on it. And maybe it did.

I first met Debrah when she was originally referred to me through the Dental Lifeline Network (DLN), a nonprofit that provides free dental care to some of the most vulnerable people in the United States.[1] Often, the DLN sends in patients who need to be cleared for a medical procedure, meaning if a dentist discovers an infection present in their mouth, they can't be cleared for surgery. Otherwise, there's a chance the oral infection could enter the bloodstream, spread the infection, complicate the procedure, and literally put the patient at risk of death, which would defeat the purpose of the surgery to begin with.

Debrah was connected to the DLN because, many years prior, she had been involved in a horrific car accident that left

---

1   The DLN organization connects people with disabilities, the elderly, or the medically fragile—people who often cannot work and therefore cannot afford adequate dental care—with dentists willing to volunteer their time and donate necessary treatments to ensure their oral health stays, well, healthy.

her with a rare condition: her abdominal wall had been permanently severed, leaving her internal organs without that added layer of protection. Now her organs lie near the surface of her skin. (Rub your belly and imagine being able to feel all the bumps and dips of your intestines.) That puts her at such a high risk for rupture that she is pretty much wheelchair-bound—her guts are literally an epidermis thickness away from the outside world. Additionally, since the accident, she had acquired numerous illnesses and developed systemic autoimmune diseases, including severe lung disease.

Unfortunately, Debrah's lung capacity had worsened over time. Her pulmonologist wanted to put her on a monthly infusion of immunosuppressants to reduce the inflammation in her body so that she'd be able to breathe better. However, before doing so, he thought (correctly) that he should have her teeth cleaned and mouth examined to make sure she wasn't fighting off any other infections. After all, it had been years since she'd been to a dentist because she didn't think it was necessary—she wasn't suffering from any piercing tooth pain or foul oral odors. If her attitude sounds familiar, make an appointment now!

So that's how she ended up in my office the first time: for a routine cleaning and a check for infection. By the time she got there, she was gasping and could hardly breathe despite carrying a tank of oxygen. During our standard diagnostic salivary tests, we discovered Debrah had elevated enzyme levels, specifically matrix metalloproteinase-8 (MMP-8) levels. (I'll discuss MMP-8 a little later in the chapter. For now, it's important to know that high levels usually suggest some kind of periodontal disease is present in the patient's mouth—that is, their gums and bones are decaying.) Additionally, an oral bacteria test showed that her mouth housed a moderate level of infectious bacteria that harms the lungs. Right, she had a specific periodontal bacteria that is associated with lung disease. She also had some carious lesions (cavities).

Once I had a fuller picture of what was going on in Debrah's mouth, I knew I had to help her or else...If her pulmonologist put her on an immunosuppressant, she wouldn't be able to fight off any kind of bug, and the infectious bacteria I found in her mouth would only worsen her gums and lung condition. I was able to put together a treatment plan that sounds simple—we cleaned her mouth and reduced the lung-destroying bacteria—but was quite complex. It included a therapeutic procedural cleaning that involved scaling and root planing to remove the tartar and plaque above and below the gumline, oral medicaments, lasers, and cavity restorations: a fancy way to say we cleaned her mouth and reduced the lung-destroying bacteria. The results were lifesaving.

Before we go any further into Debrah's story, let's talk about dental cleanings. Basically, there are two types: the cleaning everyone (should) make an appointment for every six months and the cleaning that at least half the population actually needs.

- The first is the normal cleaning you receive twice a year from a hygienist (or clinician, as many offices no longer have hygienists). That standard, normal cleaning is called dental prophylaxis, or as I like to call it, a prophy.
- The second type is called therapeutic cleaning, the scaling and root cleaning that gets below the gumline. This type is for people with a gum infection or periodontal disease.

Prophys are for healthy patients who are free of gum infection or periodontal disease. However, there is only a 50 percent chance, if you are under the age of sixty-five, that you would need this type of cleaning. If you are over that age, the chances are 30 percent.[2]

If you're paying close attention, you'll realize what those statistics are telling you: if you're under sixty-five, you have a fifty-fifty chance of needing a therapeutic cleaning; if you're over sixty-five, you have a 70 percent chance of needing one. Debrah was clearly in that 70 percent category, *and she had no symptoms to suggest that!* (Did you call your dentist yet for an appointment?)

Debrah followed up with me about a month later to discuss the side effects of her dental treatment. She was happy to tell me her lungs had improved so much that her pulmonologist said she no longer needed to get the heavy monthly infusion of immunosuppressants. To this day, Debrah is still not receiving the immunosuppressants, which is why she didn't miss a visit with me!

While I appreciate Debrah's doctor having the vision to send her for dental care before prescribing the immunosuppressants, I know that many other patients—too many—are not being given the same opportunity. Why? Because surprisingly few patients *and* physicians (including dentists) are aware of the oral-systemic link and the impact it has on overall health. Honestly, that brings me pause. I can't help but wonder how many other people out there are suffering daily from chronic diseases that just don't seem to improve despite getting medical care. How many of them *could be* helped if they were able to get the right dental testing and treatment? What if Debrah had been sent to me when she was first diagnosed with lung disease? Could we have nipped it in the bud?

I don't know any of those answers for sure, but I believe they

---

2   Eke PI, Dye B, Wei L, Thornton-Evans G, Genco R, *Prevalence of Periodontitis in Adults in the United States: 2009 and 2010,* J Dent Res, Published online 30 August 2012:1–7, doi: 10.1177/0022034512457373.

are worth thinking about. There is an enormous number of people in our nation who are chronically diseased. That means there is an enormous number of people who would feel better physically, which would help them feel better emotionally, if they received proper dental care. It is for those people that I went into the field of dentistry. And every day the number of people who could find more joy and better health in life is increasing because the health of our nation is declining.

WE ARE A SICK COUNTRY

The United States is often perceived as one of the best countries in the world. And in many ways, we are. Unfortunately, in one way we are not, and in fact, where we are sorely lagging behind our peers is in regard to our health. According to the 2019 Bloomberg Healthiest Country Index, the US, despite being the second-richest country in the world, ranks thirty-fifth out of 169 countries when it comes to being healthy![3]

The life expectancy of Americans is actually declining. According to the CDC, life expectancy in the US fell from 78.9 years in 2019 to 76.6 years in 2021.[4] Sure, COVID-19 may have had something to do with this, but realize that our peer nations didn't suffer the same decline. Proof of our poor health was painfully apparent when pandemic death rates became public. Without question, we were less able to fight off the infection to the point that, during the pandemic, our life expectancy was about five

---

3   Lee J. Miller and Wei Lu, "These Are the World's Healthiest Nations," Bloomberg, February 24, 2019, https://www.bloomberg.com/news/articles/2019-02-24/spain-tops-italy-as-world-s-healthiest-nation-while-u-s-slips.

4   "Life Expectancy in the U.S. Dropped for the Second Year in a Row in 2021," Centers for Disease Control and Prevention, last reviewed August 31, 2022, https://www.cdc.gov/nchs/pressroom/nchs_press_releases/2022/20220831.htm#:~:text=Life%20expectancy%20at%20birth%20in,its%20lowest%20level%20since%201996.

years less than the average among those countries. What good is it to live in the land of the free if you can't live to enjoy it?

We rank so low because we are sick! The CDC reports that six out of every ten Americans suffer from a chronic disease, and four out of ten suffer from more than two.[5] Compounding the seriousness of that number is the fact that, of the leading causes of death in this country, seven out of the top eight result from preventable diseases—all those diseases we wouldn't get if we'd just follow through on our New Year's resolutions. They are, listed in the order of most prevalent first:

1. Heart disease
2. Cancer
3. Chronic respiratory disease
4. Accidents
5. Stroke
6. Alzheimer's
7. Diabetes
8. Influenza and pneumonia

Not only are those conditions killing us in great numbers, but the prevalence of many of them is on the rise, too, which means we are only getting sicker.

All these stats beg the same questions: What's causing chronic disease? What's killing us? Well, the short answer is inflammation. Seven out of those eight conditions listed above are caused by inflammation. You could even say that all of them are impacted by inflammation—even accidents, which come in at number four. Most lethal accidents are caused by sleep

---

5   Centers for Disease Control and Prevention, "National Center for Chronic Disease Prevention and Health Promotion (NCCDPHP)," last reviewed March 2, 2023, https://www.cdc.gov/chronicdisease/index.htm.

apnea, which has a relationship with inflammation. We'll dive into each of those diseases and the role of inflammation in later chapters. What's important to recognize here is that it doesn't have to be this way. Inflammation can be reined in, and by doing so, overall health and well-being will increase.

WHAT LIGHTS THE FIRE OF INFLAMMATION?

In their book, *Beat the Heart Attack Gene,* authors Bradly Bale, MD, Amy Doneen, ARNP, and Lisa Collier Cool expose the health-related causes of inflammation.[6] Those causes include:

- Cariogenic bacteria (the bacteria that causes decay)
- Endodontic (tooth) abscess
- Genetics (IL-6 mutation, in particular)
- Insulin resistance (diabetes)
- Obstructive sleep apnea
- Periodontal disease
- Periodontal pathogens
- Rheumatoid arthritis (an autoimmune disease)
- Smoking and secondhand smoke
- Stress

I would add excessive alcohol, poor nutrition, and obesity to that list. Obesity is another growing problem in this country. The technical definition from the CDC for obesity is when someone's body mass index (BMI)—a number calculated from a person's weight and height—is over 30.[7] When you combine

---

6   Bradley Bale, Amy Doneen, and Lisa Collier Cool. *Beat the Heart Attack Gene: The Revolutionary Plan to Prevent Heart Disease, Stroke, and Diabetes* (Nashville: Wiley, 2014).

7   Centers for Disease Control and Prevention, "Adult BMI (Body Mass Index) Calculator," last reviewed November 3, 2020, https://www.cdc.gov/widgets/healthyliving/index.html#bmicalculator.

people who are overweight (BMI between 25 and 30) with those who are obese, a whopping 74.9 percent of us are overweight or obese! That's three-quarters of the population! (There's definitely a quarter-pounder joke in there somewhere.)

Our weight matters. There is a direct causal relationship between weight and inflammation. Fat, especially visceral fat, is considered by some to be an organ in itself, secreting inflammatory cells and hormones. Excess fat on a person's body stimulates inflammatory markers. So the heavier a person is, the more likely they will suffer from inflammation throughout the body.[8]

Then there's stress. Who isn't stressed these days, especially after surviving the pandemic and subsequent fallout? While stress cannot be avoided, it should be managed because when it's not, our health suffers. Stress triggers our bodies to be in fight-or-flight mode, which was useful thousands of years ago when we had to do things like run from lions who thought we'd make a nice meal. When fight-or-flight is triggered, our bodily processes shift into gear to create the hormones cortisol and adrenaline (among other things), which help us get the hell out of Dodge as quickly as possible.

So in the case of emergencies, fight-or-flight mode is just what we need. But it is designed to be used in short bursts to help us survive an acute situation. It is not meant to be chronically turned on like it is today from our overexposure to bad news in the media, traffic jams, inflation, and teachers sending emails about our kids. Each stressful episode just builds on the other. Our bodies keep pumping out cortisol. Over time, our digestion shuts down (including our saliva production, leading

---

8   Mohammed S. Ellulu et al., "Obesity and Inflammation: The Linking Mechanism and the Complications," *Archives of Medical Science* 13, no. 4 (2017): 851–863, https://doi.org/10.5114/aoms.2016.58928.

to dry mouth), blood sugar regulation is disrupted, cells die, and, oh yeah, inflammation. Stress kills.

Deep breath.

That was a lot to take in, I'm sure. Entire books are written on the connections between weight and stress and health. I kept it to a minimum to fit it within this book. We will now be looking specifically at inflammatory responses, what causes inflammation, and how it affects disease.

Did you know that your teeth are organs too? They are living and are composed of tissue, blood supply, and a nerve. So when our bodies are stressed out, it affects our teeth and vice versa. Tooth infections, if not treated, cause chronic inflammation, which puts our bodies into a chronic state of fight-or-flight. If your liver stops working, you are quickly placed on an organ transplant list to replace that vital organ. Why are we not as concerned about replacing our tooth organs, knowing how vital they are to our overall health?

INFLAMMATION IS EXPENSIVE!

I realize I've filled the beginning of this book with data and statistics. I promise the rest of it will not be so math-dense, but before we end this chapter, we need to look at what all this inflammation-induced chronic disease is costing us as a nation and individually. Personal healthcare expenditures, per capita, were $11,582 in 2019. By now it probably isn't a surprise to learn that number is an increase over what was spent in the past. In fact, it's more than double the $4,119 per capita cost in 2000. Those totals, when extrapolated to the entire population, come to $1.2 trillion in 2000 and $3.8 trillion spent on personal healthcare in 2019![9]

But perhaps the biggest cost of inflammation is the very personal consequence to a person's health. The good news here, though, is that nearly all inflammation is preventable. And that prevention starts in the mouth.

Many people may not be surprised to read that oral bacteria is bad for their health. After all, anyone with an artificial joint or a heart problem must take an antibiotic every time they go to the dentist. But it's shocking how many Americans are completely unaware that they can improve their health by taking care of their mouth (the story of my career).

Perhaps that's because most Americans see dental care as mostly a luxury and a part-time, on-occasion need (also the story of my career). They assume dentists exist to clean their teeth, fix their smile with braces or bleaching, and fill cavities or pull out wisdom teeth. That limited opinion of dental care might be why not everyone visits a dentist every year. And for some bizarre reason I just don't understand, the older we get, the less likely we'll make those routine-care appointments. Our seniors are more at risk for dental disease for a number of reasons. Additionally, they often suffer from comorbidities of heart disease, diabetes, dementia, lung disease, and cancer and would greatly benefit from dental care.

However, while routine exams and cleanings, braces, and cavity fillings are all important procedures, as seen in Debrah's story, dentists can play a much larger role in a person's overall physical health. Dentists now have diagnostic tests and technologies that can help uncover the causes of many diseases—including the chronic ones listed earlier. Even better,

---

9 "Health Expenditures," Centers for Disease Control and Prevention, last reviewed February 23, 2023, https://www.cdc.gov/nchs/fastats/health-expenditures.htm.

they can effectively respond to those causes, stop them in their tracks, and prevent or reverse the disease states. They can examine your mouth, discover what could be making you sick (or will make you sick later if left unattended), and then target any infection or inflammation and treat it to improve your oral health, which, in turn, will improve your overall health.

If everyone went and received the appropriate dental care they truly need, they would not only improve their personal health, but they might also discover their pocketbooks have a little extra in them too. In fact, patients with chronic diseases who undergo dental or periodontal treatment can save thousands of dollars each year.

- Stroke patients save an average of $5,681 and have 21.2 percent fewer hospitalizations.
- Patients with heart disease save $1,090 and have 28.6 percent fewer hospitalizations.
- Diabetes patients each save about $2,850 and have 39.4 percent fewer hospitalizations.
- Pregnant patients save $2,433.[10]

In short, if you want to save money, be healthier, and live longer, go see your dentist! Your mouth is probably what's causing or feeding your health problems.

To get a better understanding of how that works, let's look at the role of your mouth and inflammation in your body.

10   Marjorie K. Jeffcoat, et al., "Impact of Periodontal Therapy on General Health: Evidence from Insurance Data for Five Systemic Conditions," American Jorunal of Preventative Medicine, June 18, 2014, DOI: https://doi.org/10.1016/j.amepre.2014.04.001.

CHAPTER 2

Your Mouth Is Feeding the Problem

"YEAH, I KNOW YOU. YOU SAVED MY LIFE."

Kelly had just started working for me at one of my satellite offices as our treatment coordinator. But when I went out to introduce myself to her on her first day, I learned we'd already met before. As it turned out, she had been a patient of mine some years back. It had been so long that I'd forgotten about our encounter. I felt a little guilty about that, but thankfully, she didn't hold a grudge. After I apologized for my forgetfulness, she filled me in on her amazing journey.

Kelly had suffered from a lifetime of bleeding gums, and every dentist she'd had since childhood simply told her to "brush and floss better." So she did. In fact, she had better oral hygiene than most people, and in her efforts to find another opinion, Kelly wound up at my office.

As soon as she got into my chair, I knew something was wrong. Her gums were flaming red and painfully swollen. Normally when people have such severe inflammation, there's an extreme amount of plaque and tartar on the teeth, but Kelly's were spotless; she took immaculate care of her mouth. I knew something was up.

We performed a salivary test to check for bacteria, a DNA test to scan for the interleukin 6 (IL-6) gene mutation, and a perio fit test to see her MMP-8 enzyme levels. (I'll discuss all of these in detail later, but for now, just know that they help determine inflammation levels and how oral bacteria is affecting the rest of the body.) Her results were off the freaking charts. When MMP-8 levels are over twenty nanograms per milliliter (ng/mL), bacteria can enter the bloodstream freely; anything over fifty is considered severe. *Kelly's levels were over one hundred.* She also tested positive for the IL-6 mutation, which is a gene that upregulates (that is, turns on in a not-sexy way) the immune system. That sounds great in theory, but it also means you are more prone to inflammatory reactions.

Again, this was all highly irregular without the presence of etiology (that is, evidence of disease) or of plaque and tartar. We cleaned her mouth with nonsurgical periodontal therapy, I urged her to tell her primary care physician about all we had found and to have a complete physical and blood workup, and I put her on a two-month recall. I never heard back from her. That had been the end of the story until now.

It turned out she took my advice and went to see her doctor. After much blood work and many tests and X-rays, they found she had systemic endometriosis. The disorder had even spread to her respiratory system, causing lesions on her lungs. To top it off, she had developed polycystic ovarian syndrome (PCOS)— all due to the inflammation in her body that wasn't obvious except in her mouth. Fortunately, the medical treatment for her endometriosis and PCOS proved effective, and all issues were resolved, including her inflamed gums. Kelly now stood before me completely healed because her mouth told me she had a problem. (She now gets her teeth cleaned at the office where she works.)

"You saved my life. I wanted to come work for you and help others the way you helped me."

I was speechless.

IT'S ALL ABOUT THE INFLAMMATION, BABY!

In Chapter 1, I discussed some of the causes of inflammation in our bodies, but I didn't explain how inflammation happens or why. The thing is, a little bit of inflammation is something you actually *want* to happen every now and then (unlike that visit from your crazy political uncle you have to endure every year at Thanksgiving). Inflammation is the body's response to attack and injury. Think back to when you were a child, learning how hot the stove was. "Don't touch it—it'll burn you!" said Mom, but you did it anyway. That hot, swollen, painful red hand was the result of inflammation. On the psychological level, inflammation is your body's way of saying, "Hey, listen to your mother" and giving you a reason to never injure yourself like that again. But on the biological level, wonders are occurring.

The goal of inflammation is to protect and heal our bodies. When our bodies are subjected to invasion (e.g., a bacterial or viral infection) or injury, our immune system releases an army of white blood cells to fight and kill off the invading agents, allowing any damaged tissues to be healed. In addition, the body can also release proteins, called cytokines, that stimulate the release of additional inflammatory cells as needed. Think of cytokines as the reserve forces.

After the immune system releases white blood cells (WBCs) during an invasion, the body also releases an activated form of an enzyme called MMP-8. Essentially, MMP-8 acts as a pair of scissors that cuts apart the connections between cells, which is what allows the WBC army to blaze a trail through the tissues and reach the intruder.

Inflammation results when all the fluids necessary to carry the WBCs and MMP-8 arrive at the site of the attack. So, really, inflammation is necessary for healing—if you don't become inflamed, that means your WBCs aren't getting to ground zero, where they need to be, and the bacteria are partying away.

While inflammation is helpful in acute situations, it becomes detrimental over an extended amount of time because it can cause or exacerbate other diseases in our bodies, as I spoke about in the previous chapter. Which begs the question: What causes chronic inflammation?

THE MOUTH-BODY CONNECTION

Chronic inflammation means your body is in a constant state of attacking something. The body is always activated and working—it never gets to rest. Frequently, the something it's so busy fighting is bacteria. And if we follow the chain of investigation here, that means we need to look at where the bacteria come from. The answer to that is often—you guessed it—your mouth.

Modern medicine tends to focus solely on the internal systems (heart, stomach, colon, brain, lungs, etc.) and view them as independent organs instead of an integrated system, missing the bigger picture of how individual systems are affected by the overall bodily environment—a "missing the body through the organs" type of mistake, if you will. That oversight is entirely understandable; if the heart stops working, look at the heart. *Who looks at the mouth?* No one. No one really looks at the mouth in the same way, right? It's counterintuitive, I know, but they should because our mouths are a gateway for bacteria to enter and circulate in the body. Some of the bacteria make their way inside because you swallow them, but much more is absorbed through your gums.

Our gums are essentially made from the same tissue as our skin. As you've heard since middle school, our skin is our largest organ (sorry, guys) and the primary defense in protecting our insides from the outside. Your gums are tasked with the same job, and part of their defensive armory is the oral microbiome.

You may be familiar with the microbiome associated with your gut—basically, it's the billions of microorganisms that line your intestines. That microbiome is made from all the friendly bacteria we ingest, like the good kind we get from the probiotics in yogurt and the bad kind we get from other people and unhealthy foods—the ones you've been told all your life not to eat: sugar, processed stuff, things with artificial colors and crap. What you may not be familiar with is your oral microbiome, which is made up of all the healthy and unhealthy bacteria in your mouth.

While your mouth is small in comparison to your intestinal tract, don't be fooled into thinking it plays a small role in your health. The oral microbiome is the second-largest microbiome in the human body, but it is often the first line of defense against bad bacteria. Most everyone is familiar with gut health: make sure the good bacteria outweigh the bad. This same principle *should* be applied to the mouth as well, and unlike what they say about dogs, our mouths are the dirtiest parts of us humans.

Because our society has become obsessed with overcleaning and sterilization, our mouths are in a constant state of dysbiosis (microflora disruption). We'll get into problems with overcleaning later in the book, but for now, realize that certain mouthwashes and toothpastes will tip the balance of good and bad oral bacteria over to the dark side of the force, leading to disease. Meanwhile, bacteria existing in the month is a widely known fact; cariogenic bacteria causing cavities and abscesses from infected root canals (endodontic abscesses) is common knowledge. What may not be common knowledge is when bacteria isn't properly handled and eliminated, the damage goes beyond the teeth. It causes disease, and it kick-starts an inflammatory response.

If you develop chronic inflammation because of the bacteria present in your mouth, then you will be in a perpetual state of MMP-8 cutting through the cells in your gum tissue—you'll be a "perforated person" (I love alliteration). The level of activated MMP-8 is in direct correlation with the level of inflammation in our bodies—meaning the more inflammation, the more cells are separated, which leaves a wide-open gate for bacteria to enter your body.

In the mouth, this issue is known as "leaky gums." Chronic inflammation of our mouths deteriorates our gums (which, remember, is like skin: the primary immune barrier) and lets the numerous bad bacteria pour on in and circulate through our body; it's basically an open-borders policy. This is the exact same issue as what occurs in the more widely known "leaky gut syndrome," where the intestines become permeable and allow toxins from waste (poop) to leak into our bodies (gross).

Symptoms of leaky gut are evident: diarrhea, constipation, bloating, gas, and abdominal discomfort. The stark difference between leaky gut and gums is that you often can't *feel* leaky gums. (Thankfully, nowadays, dentists can test for leaky gums. Even if your dentist doesn't have this test, they'll have other ways of detecting leaky gums.) But just because you can't feel the problem doesn't mean there isn't one. Without you even knowing it, you can have gaping passageways between the cells in your gums allowing harmful entities (like bad bacteria) to pass through and invade the rest of your body.

You may have already figured this out, but it's for this reason that physicians prescribe premedication. Doctors have some patients take antibiotics prior to dental treatment because they know that whatever a person puts in their mouth will wind up in their bloodstream. That's why you need antibiotic premedication when you go to the dentist for cleanings if you have a compromised immune system, unrepaired congenital heart defects, heart valve replacements, and even some joint replacements: in the event that the cleaning releases bacteria into your bloodstream, the antibiotics can protect you from getting sick.

MORE THAN GENETICS

At this point you may be questioning where genetics fits in. After all, everyone knows someone whose father had a heart attack in his midfifties, as did their grandfather and great-grandfather. And no doubt, genetics does play a role in how well our bodies function; this is easily observed in familial diseases. However, intrinsic biological characteristics are only half the story. In fact, less than 20 percent of all diseases are caused by genetics.[11] The remaining 80 percent are influenced by epigenetics: the environment and behaviors that change our gene expression. Do you know which major player causes those changes? Yep, it's inflammation. Inflammation that is rooted in the mouth.

You see, we are born basically sterilized. As infants, being kissed and placing everything from toys to shoes in our mouths,

---

11   Stephen M. Rappaport, "Genetic Factors Are Not the Major Causes of Chronic Diseases," *PLoS ONE* 11, no. 4 (2016): e0154387, https://doi.org/10.1371/journal.pone.0154387.

we pick up seven hundred plus strains of bacteria (yeah, gross, again). That is to say, all of our bacteria are *acquired* (our first introduction to bacteria is coming through the birthing canal). As we'll discuss further in this chapter, there are eleven main types of bacteria that cause periodontal/oral disease, and naturally, groups of people in one location (like a family) will share common bacteria. What I'm saying is that passed-down diseases are often caused by passed-down bacteria, not genes.

Because of that, if I have a patient who tests positive for harmful bacteria in their salivary test, I will ask them to bring their spouse and children into my practice for further testing. Almost unerringly, their other family members will test positive for the bacteria as well. From there, I explain how if I treat only one family member, they will become reinfected once they share a kiss, utensil, or food with each other, and the cycle of disease will continue. That is how genes and learned familial behaviors (e.g., smoking, poor diet) create a perfect and perpetuating storm of inflammation and disease. So while genetics can play a role, it's more of a side character to the mouth as the lead.

FROM TOP TO BOTTOM

One of the major issues I face in educating people about the mouth-body connection is that somewhere in history a disconnection was made between what happens in someone's mouth and what is considered normal. For instance, if you were to lightly scratch an itch, only to then look down and see your forearm dripping with blood, you'd immediately think something was wrong and probably schedule an appointment with a dermatologist right away. But time and time again, I have patients whose gums start to bleed when they brush their teeth, and when I question them on this obvious problem, the response is always the same: "Oh, it's normal. I've been like that since I was a kid." Why on earth would anyone think that the gentle bristle of a toothbrush causing bleeding is normal? It's bass-ackwards and needs to be corrected. If there's bleeding, there's an infection and overgrowth of harmful bacteria. If it "always happens," that means you've had a lifetime of chronic inflammation. No one should be okay with their gums bleeding, ever!

Of the seven hundred plus bacteria found in the mouth (once again, gross), there are eleven specific strains that are the main causes of periodontal disease and also affect systemic disease. These are:

- *Treponema denticola* (Td)
- *Prevotella intermedia* (Pi)
- *Actinobacillus actinomycetemcomitans* (Aa)
- *Eikenella corrodens* (Ec)
- *Fusobacterium nucleatum/periodontal* (Fn)
- *Eubacterium nodatum* (En)
- *Campylobacter rectus* (Cr)
- *Tannerella forsythia* (Tf)
- *Capnocytophaga* (Cs)
- *Peptostreptococcus micros* (Pm)
- *Porphyromonas gingivalis* (Pg)

All of these have been linked to health issues ranging from cancer to maternity complications and tied to the top eight deadly diseases mentioned in Chapter 1.

Six of these eleven bacteria are resistant to conventional forms of dental treatment (that is, regular and periodontal cleanings). So when patients come in and "only want their regular cleaning," over 50 percent of the bacteria that cause life-threatening diseases are left untreated (and remember the stats from Chapter 1: 50 to 70 percent of the people reading this book need more than that standard cleaning). This is why people will nonchalantly say their gums have bled all their lives—*they have had a bacterial infection that has never been treated.* Medicaments are needed to address those other six, which are not part of a standard cleaning.

BUT WAIT, THERE'S MORE!

Also not part of a standard cleaning is a check for abscesses— that is why it is important to also get a dental exam. When a tooth dies, the nerves and blood vessels in the tooth die as well (called necrosis). This releases bacterial excrement (yes, bacteria poops) and toxins into the connected bony space, which leads to infection and creates a pocket of pus called an abscess, which is often—surprisingly—not painful. The lack of pain occurs when the abscess is able to drain toxins into the body (it swells when it cannot drain, and that's when you feel the pain). Your body doesn't want the toxins and kicks an immune response into gear. Left unchecked, the drainage from the abscess can cause chronic inflammation and lead to other complications. Meanwhile, because of the lack of pain, the sufferer is at a loss to explain the inflammation. They often do not know they have systemic inflammation from an abscess. In this way, an abscess can be a silent killer.

Abscesses can also be formed within the gum tissues by gum disease bacteria. Regardless of the cause, though, an abscess can be a real danger. Left untreated, an abscess can spread to the bone (osteomyelitis), to the surrounding soft tissues (cellulitis of the muscles/fat), or to the sinus and pharyngeal space, causing breathing issues. At worst, it spreads to the brain, causing death (you don't want a bacterial infection of the brain—it ain't pretty). Without swelling or pain (or with a lifetime of symptom normalization) the problem persists and develops unknowingly. Fortunately, abscesses show up on dental X-rays. Again, regular checkups are encouraged.

Unfelt abscesses are common in teeth previously treated with root canals, which is why many holistic clinicians advise that such teeth be removed or the procedure be avoided altogether (especially in the presence of chronic illness).[12] Once a tooth has had a root canal, it is essentially dead—there's no nerve or blood supply to the tooth. So if an infection recurs, the patient often doesn't feel it because the tooth is lifeless. A dead tooth has no blood supply or immune system to protect itself, so an abscess forms and persists. These teeth are also at an increased risk of recurrent decay and bone loss because they are lacking a lifeline. If your immune system is busy fighting a constant stream of infection from an abscess in your jawbone, it will not be able to address other issues in your body as they come—God forbid that your immune system be fighting a latent mouth infection when it could be fighting off cancer! Basically, by giving some focus to oral health, you help your body help itself.

In short: if your gums are bleeding while you're brushing or flossing, it's not normal. And if you are waking up with blood in your mouth or have loose teeth, that's *definitely* not normal. For both, you need to see a dentist right away. These symptoms, along with itchy gums, painful eating, and particularly bad breath, are signs of gum disease and are a likely cause of other health issues you are experiencing.

---

12   I'm not advocating for or against root canals but merely providing information; plenty of patients have root canals that perform as expected, but we can't deny the associated risks.

KNOWLEDGE IS POWER

Ever hear about someone dying from a tooth infection? I was speaking with a friend recently (outside of the dental care industry) who told me how one of their family members wound up with a heart infection after a dental procedure. They had never understood the connection, but once I explained the systemic nature of our bodies and how bacterial infections can travel via the circulatory system, it all became obvious to her—but this information is relatively new to most people. So they don't give it the attention they should.

Two hundred years ago, it was a different story. Back then, a tooth infection was a leading cause of death. While it's rare to die from a tooth infection today, there is still a one in one thousand chance of the worst happening from such an infection, which means you need to pay attention to this! Are you thinking, "Dr. Lee, isn't this a bit alarmist for a one out of a thousand chance?" Well, to put that in perspective, we all know the importance of having smoke detectors in our homes, but the chance of dying from a fire is only about one in fifteen hundred (death by tooth infection is one and a half times more likely).[13] A one in one thousand chance happens more often than you'd think, and when the outcome is such an extreme as potential death, it's wise to take it seriously.

Luckily, Kelly found this knowledge in her twenties, but there are plenty of others who never do and spend their lives needlessly suffering. I applaud your willingness to learn and seek out answers by picking up this book; you're taking the initial steps in your healing journey. And now that you understand how your mouth is connected to disease in general, let's look at some specific health concerns and how they are impacted by oral health.

---

13 National Safety Council, "Odds of Dying," NSC Injury Facts, accessed December 14, 2022, https://injuryfacts.nsc.org/all-injuries/preventable-death-overview/odds-of-dying.

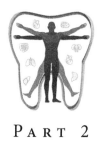

THE MOUTH-BODY CONNECTION— DISEASES AND AILMENTS

CHAPTER 3

The Heart That Kills

JON WAS A NEW PATIENT AT MY PRACTICE, SO, AS WITH all my new patients, I conducted a new-patient interview to see why he'd come in that day and also to get a read on where he was in understanding the mouth-body connection. (I've found that *no one* likes to be preached at, and I do not force information onto patients.) He was the perfect specimen of health—a handsome, fit middle-aged man. He had no ailments common to men of his age, was lean, and exercised on the regular. It was easy to see that he took good care of himself and that he cared about his health.

"So, how can I help you today?" I asked.

"Oh, you know, just here to get my regular checkup and cleaning. 'Check the box' as they say."

"Sounds great," I nodded. "Let's start with the X-rays."

I took a cone-beam computed technology (CBCT) scan and digital X-rays and performed a full dental exam. With how Jon prided himself on his health and his lack of any symptoms, I didn't expect to find much. However, because of my experience, I knew that anything was possible and did a thorough checkup.

After finishing the exam, I came back to him with the results. We were both shocked, to say the least.

"Jon, your mouth is infected…everywhere."

"What does that mean?"

"You have periodontal disease."

He recoiled. "But I feel fine! I don't even have bad breath!"

"And your root canals…they've abscessed."

Jon was in disbelief. Despite his lack of pain and relatively clean teeth, he had advanced gum disease and sacs of pus in his jawbone. I went on to explain to him the connection between our mouths and bodies, how abscesses can be present and harmful without pain, and the dangers of chronic inflammation, as well as how we should fix these issues now.

"But I don't have any pain. And I don't have high blood pressure or cholesterol or any of the other stuff you said."

"Even still, the infection is there and causing issues. Your body is constantly fighting it off. Even as we speak."

"Well," he rationalized, "if it was hurting, I'd guess I'd do something about it. I can't pay for it right now anyway. I'm trying to put my kids through college and still have a few at home too. Maybe when my finances are a little less tight, I'll come back."

We finished up, and Jon went back to his life, and I to my other patients. A year or two went by, and there was no word from Jon. I expected that he'd either moved or was turned off by my holistic mumbo jumbo and had found another doctor. But much to my surprise, I found Jon sitting in my waiting room one bright summer morning.

"Hi, Jon! Back for another cleaning, I presume?"

"No, I want to take care of those issues you found years back."

"Okay," I nodded. "Why now? Did your kids make it out of college?"

"Actually," he said, shifting his gaze to me, "I had a heart attack."

Jon went on to explain how, recently, he had been working out, and his chest had suddenly become tight. It scared him so much that he immediately drove himself to the hospital. After they took their tests, the doctors confirmed that Jon was having a heart attack, and the cardiologist ordered a complete workup on him to find the cause. Everything looked fine—his cholesterol was a little high, but it was nothing that should have caused a heart attack. After finding no clear reason for the attack, Jon's doctor suggested that the issue could have originated from his mouth.

"Naturally, I thought of you. And all you had told me about gum disease and those abscesses."

I was glad he had remembered.

"I want to be around for my kids—they need me. So I'd like to get this problem solved as soon as possible. I'll figure out the finances."

Jon was a classic example of our traditional understanding of heart health: eating bad foods leads to clogged arteries leads to blockage leads to dropping dead from a heart attack. Later, I'll extrapolate further, but for now, know that, basically, this notion is completely disproved by modern medicine. In fact, our bodies can miraculously heal themselves (similar to how the liver can regenerate despite the daily dump of toxins we give it), and (spoiler alert) heart attacks are caused by inflammation, which, as you now know, directly correlates to oral health. So a healthy mouth can make for a healthy heart.

Jon was also the embodiment of our typical response to health issues: "If it ain't broke, don't fix it." Continually, I warn my patients that their current, seemingly asymptomatic mouth problems will create health complications, and continually, my patients put it off because it isn't an issue at the moment—it's a "we'll cross that bridge when we get there" type of attitude. But the truth is they've already smashed through the "Bridge Out Ahead" sign.

Proactivity is vital in this arena. If you don't heed the warning signs of poor oral hygiene, you could end up in the same place as Jon, or worse. Many signs of disease do not hurt or have symptoms. High blood pressure, for example, doesn't hurt until you have a heart attack. Periodontal disease doesn't hurt until you have an abscess or your tooth falls out. Cancer does not hurt until the very end. Pain cannot be the only thing we pay attention to when deciding if we should take action.

This is precisely why I'm writing this book: to educate and support healthier living. In this chapter, I'll do so with an overview of heart disease and how your mouth's health impacts it.

(DON'T) BE STILL, MY HEART

You can live without food for weeks, water for days, and air for minutes. But how long can you live without blood? (Hint, hint, it's *a lot* shorter.) Being that your heart supplies that blood, it's wholly responsible for keeping you alive. So it's useful to know how the heart works and what can harm it.

The heart is made up of four different chambers. Blood comes in, gets pumped through chamber by chamber, and exits to circulate throughout the rest of the body, carrying with it the oxygen needed for all of our tissues and organs to function. Long story short, your brain, lungs, muscles, and everything in your body depends upon your heart passing along the blood needed to survive, and anything that threatens the heart from doing such threatens you as a whole.

Heart disease is the broad term that encompasses anything

that impedes the heart's function; this comes with a smorgasbord of ailments. The main complications are coronary artery disease (damage to the heart's blood vessels), hypertension (overly high pressure in the blood vessels), myocardial infarction (acute necrosis of heart tissue), congestive heart failure (heart not pumping enough blood to the body), and arrhythmia (irregularity in the heart's electrical system, causing it not to fire correctly). Common causes of heart disease are atherosclerosis (fatty plaques building up in the vessels), high blood pressure, high cholesterol, smoking, obesity, diabetes, periodontal disease, and obstructive sleep apnea. Basically, heart disease is anything that can stop blood from entering the heart, cause the heart itself to function improperly, or impede blood from traveling away from the heart.

A quick note about heart attacks: the commonly held belief is that heart attacks occur when plaque formations build up over time in our arteries and close off the blood vessel. *Wrong.* Autopsies show that our hearts can form new blood vessels that bypass obstacles through a process called angiogenesis (Latin for "detour: road closed ahead"). Plaque, while it does weaken the vessel wall it's attached to, it can silently exist as long as nothing disturbs it; the body compensates for its presence. However, acute inflammation disrupts plaque and dislodges it, tearing the vessel open—not good!

Because the insides of our vessels are sticky, when plaque "pops" off an artery, it takes arterial tissue with it, ripping open the vessel and causing it to bleed. Once the vessel is torn, the body secretes certain proteins to stop the bleeding, and it's this clot that stops the blood flow to the heart, scientifically known as a *myocardial infarction.*

All that to say, while having a poor diet and high choles-terol is damaging and certainly not recommended, these are not the only causes of heart attacks. Bacterial infections, often originating from the mouth, can cause heart attacks as well by initiating inflammation.

THE QUICKEST WAY TO A MAN'S HEART IS THROUGH HIS MOUTH

In their medical studies, Bradley Bale, MD, Amy Doneen, ARNP, and Lisa Collier Cool (authors of *Beat the Heart Attack Gene*) found that 50 percent of all heart attacks and strokes are caused by oral bacteria (with Aa and Pg primarily and Tf, Td, and Fn being associated).[14] A recent study discovered 100 percent of patients with cardiovascular disease had Pg colonizing in their arteries![15] Even more astounding, of the people who die from a heart attack or stroke, researchers found that 70 percent of the fatal blood clots were made of the same oral bacteria. That is to say, not only is poor oral hygiene strongly linked to heart attacks and strokes, but it also causes them to be more deadly. *Yikes!*

The mechanics behind this are like so: with chronic inflam-mation in our mouth, we see the previously discussed leaky gum syndrome per our frenemy MMP-8. Openings form in the gums, and one (or more) of the five bacteria linked to heart disease listed above enter the bloodstream. Think of your blood vessels (arteries, veins, etc.) as long balloons, like the ones you make balloon animals with. You want the insides of the balloons to be clean and wide to allow blood to flow smoothly. When suffering a bacterial infection, these bacteria cause the interior

---

14   Bale, Doneen, and Cool, *Beat the Heart Attack Gene.*

15   Stephen S. Dominy et al., "*Porphyromonas gingivalis* in Alzheimer's Disease Brains: Evidence for Disease Causation and Treatment with Small-Molecule Inhibitors," *Science Advances* 5, no. 1 (January 2019): eaau3333, https://doi.org/10.1126/sciadv.aau3333.

walls to become sticky. Then the cholesterol, fatty acids, plaques, and so on passing through your circulatory system get hung up and build a lining in your blood vessels, causing them to shrink in volume. Pg and Aa accelerate this process and the inflammatory response, creating clogged and inflamed vessels with a high probability of ripping—asty!

IT DOESN'T HAVE TO BE THAT WAY

Ever heard the one where an uncle goes to the dentist to get a deep cleaning, only to die of a heart attack hours later? It's no urban legend. It's called bacteremia. Bacteremia is the condition where bacteria enter the bloodstream (via aMMP-8) and circulate through the body. This happens more than you think. In fact, 40 percent of the bacteria in your mouth enters your bloodstream during periodontal cleanings, 35–60 percent with tooth extractions, 23 percent with daily brushing, and 17 percent while eating.[16] It's a bit of a "damned if you do, damned if you don't" type of situation. This doesn't mean you get to avoid the dentist. It's best to see your dentist regularly so they can keep the overall quantity of bacteria down to prevent these issues.

If you've read this far, the connection between gum and heart disease isn't something new to you. However, it wasn't until a recent study that the American Heart Association was able to say that gum disease is *causal* to heart disease.[17] In this study, arterial plaque was taken from patients and analyzed. When Pg and Aa were found in every sample, a direct link was

16 Peter B. Lockhart, et al., "Bacteremia Associated With Toothbrushing and Dental Extraction," *Circulation* 117, no. 24 (June 9, 2008): 3118–3125, https://doi.org/10.1161/CIRCULATIONAHA.107.758524.

17 Bradley Field Bale, Amy Lynn Doneen, and David John Vigerust, "High-Risk Periodontal Pathogens Contribute to the Pathogenesis of Atherosclerosis," *Postgraduate Medical Journal* 93, no. 1098 (April 2017): 215–220, https://doi.org/10.1136/postgradmedj-2016-134279.

made. Now when dentists discover gum disease in their patients' mouths, they can insist on treating it to prevent heart disease.

Since the American Heart Association's declaration, many more people have become aware of the link between gum and heart disease. However, now when considering their oral health, many people tend to *only* attribute gum disease to heart disease, saying, "Well, I don't have gum disease. So I needn't worry about my heart." This is not the case. *Streptococcus mutans* (the bacteria that causes cavities) is also the bacteria responsible for 50 percent of infective endocarditis cases (heart infection). So patients should also worry about cavities as well as gum disease when it comes to heart health.

The mistake here is that while the cavity-causing bacteria are not "in the gums," they are still in the mouth. We *still* get the immune response with MMP-8. Then we get leaky gums, and the bacteria gets to the heart, and you know the rest…Recognize that the whole of the body's health depends on the *whole* of the mouth's health.

In my practice, I go over family medical histories and look for high blood pressure, high cholesterol, heart attacks, A-fib (arrhythmia), and strokes (as well as other issues that we'll get into later, such as diabetes and dementia). I especially do this if the patient is young as most of these health issues have around a ten-year "ramp period" where the disease is changing the body but the effects are below the threshold where medicine would diagnose it as a condition. Obviously, most twenty-five-year-olds won't have had a heart attack or high blood pressure, but that does not mean they are not at risk. If their salivary test comes back showing positive for one of these bacteria, I start asking about their family's history with heart health and inflammation. Their answers give insight into the patient's risk and disease progression.

THE MOUTH-HEART CONNECTION

The connection between oral and heart health is clearly evident. It saddens me to see how many people put off their oral health only to continue suffering from some seemingly unrelated condition or, worse, have a heart attack, as Jon did! Jon was lucky; his heart attack could have been much worse, even fatal. Fortunately, he survived and saw the importance of all I'm sharing with you. Don't be like Jon and wait for an extreme circumstance to care for your mouth. *An ounce of prevention*, as they say.

But this part of the book is about the connection between the mouth and the whole body, not just the heart. Let's move on and look at how what's in the mouth can cause diabetes—and no, I'm not just talking about the leftover birthday cake you had for breakfast.

CHAPTER 4

Diabetes: It's Not Just for Juveniles Anymore

LET'S TALK ABOUT SUE. SUE WAS AROUND SEVENTY AND had been a patient of mine for more than ten years. I knew she was suffering from uncontrolled diabetes—her A1C score ranged from ten to fourteen (I'll explain why that's a bad thing later in the chapter). Because her extreme diabetes caused excessive blood sugar levels, Sue's teeth had rampant decay. Her tongue was pale, bald, and cracked, and it burned with pain. Her gums bled and were so sensitive that she avoided brushing and flossing despite the abstinence exacerbating the problem (during checkups she would wince in pain with the lightest touch). As is typical for many diabetics in that state, she had angular cheilitis (painful sores at the corner of the mouth), xerostomia (unusually dry mouth), thrush (fungal overgrowth in the mouth), and no will to live. Often, during our visits, she would tell me, "I'm ready to die, doctor. I'm just ready to die." Sue had been suffering for a *long* time.

At the request of her diabetologist, we focused on staving off infection in her mouth, but it was a constant uphill battle. We would clean her gums and restore cavities, only for her to return a few months later with even more cavities forming around the recent fillings. The option of pulling her teeth was considered, but we had strong reservations due to her blood sugar levels measuring as high as 200 or 300 when she was at our office.[18] Such high blood sugar levels drastically raise the odds of developing postsurgical infections, delay healing, and even increase the risk of the patient going into a diabetic coma. There was little we could do for her ever-diminishing quality of life.

Push did come to shove, and there were a few teeth we were forced to extract. Luckily, my specialist is world-class, and Sue managed to avoid any post-op infections. But nothing was done to actually *solve* her problem, and the decay continued. Eventually, all her teeth became nonrestorable, and she was at high risk of abscess. We had to pull *all* her teeth. It was truly a spot between a rock and a hard place.

If I didn't pull the teeth, it was only a matter of time before she would contract a severe tooth infection that could end up killing her. Normally, we'd give dentures to a patient in such a situation. However, I knew Sue wouldn't tolerate wearing dentures; with her sensitive gums, it would be like having sandpaper rubbing on her soft tissues. She didn't need that kind of pain. This left one option: implants—a risky move. With her medical history of high blood sugar, Sue could wind up in a coma or even die. But it was either have this operation or do nothing, which would lead to the same fate. Sue understood the risks and decided to proceed.

A periodontist, Sue's diabetologist, and I came up with a

---

18   Blood sugar in the United States is measured in milligrams per deciliter of blood. A healthy adult's blood sugar is usually less than 100 if that person hasn't recently eaten. It can go as high as 110 if they are tested shortly after ingesting foods containing carbohydrates.

treatment plan. We administered a salivary test to determine what exact bacteria were in Sue's mouth and which antibiotics to give her ahead of the procedure. She was allergic to many antibiotics, so that was another layer of difficulty we had to contend with. We gave her an antimicrobial mouthwash and also put her on an anti-inflammatory medication called Periostat. Periostat is a minocycline antibiotic that's administered at a dosage below the antibiotic threshold—meaning it doesn't have antibiotic properties and only inhibits inflammation. Periostat was used instead of the typical inflammation-fighting steroid due to the fact that steroids increase the risk of infection (not to mention also that steroids increase blood sugar levels, and we had *enough* of that already). We then scheduled the procedure, removed all her teeth, and replaced them with implants.

I saw Sue for her follow-up a month later. Her angular cheilitis had resolved, her weight was normalizing, and her A1C was below 8 percent. Needless to say, we celebrated. Even Sue's endocrinologist reached out to me, thanking me for seeing the connection between her oral health and her diabetes and for my help in getting her health stabilized. While we're not out of the woods yet (Sue still has end-stage diabetes), her mouth isn't in pain anymore, and she can eat the healthy foods that are helping her disease. That is to say, she's a hell of a lot healthier.

Unfortunately, Sue isn't the only diabetic to have oral health problems. Let's get a clear understanding of what diabetes is, how it affects the body, and how the mouth is connected to it.

AN INTRODUCTION TO DIABETES

As heart disease is the disease of the vessels of the heart, diabetes is the disease of the blood vessels of the body. As many people know, diabetes is caused by impaired glucose control, meaning the body cannot produce enough insulin, or the body stops responding to insulin, to keep blood sugar numbers within a normal range. We measure the amount of blood sugar in your system with finger-pricking tests or with an A1C test.

If you are already struggling with insulin resistance, you likely know exactly what an HbA1c means. But for those of you who don't, an A1C test measures the average amount of sugar in a person's blood over a three-month time frame. Hemoglobin is a protein found in red blood cells. When sugar is present in your blood, it binds to hemoglobin. Healthy individuals have little sugar bound to their hemoglobin, while diabetics have several sugars bound. So basically, an A1C test tells us how much sugar is free-floating in our blood. But this is more than the finger pick that you used to watch your grandmother perform; that test measures blood glucose at that moment in time. An A1C test measures the average hemoglobin levels across three months. Levels lower than 5.7 percent are normal, levels ranging from 5.7 percent to 6.4 percent are considered prediabetic, and levels above 6.5 percent show a positive test for diabetes.

One of the problems with excess sugar in our blood is that it acts like shards of glass in our blood vessels. That means, with high A1C levels, there are hundreds of thousands of pieces of "broken glass" cruising through our circulatory system, scraping their jagged edges along the walls of our blood vessels (if that doesn't make you cringe, I don't know what will). This mechanical damage alerts our body to mount an inflammatory response—one that doesn't end until blood sugar levels are normalized.

High blood sugar leads to vascular inflammation and over time impedes blood flow. Our teeth have a blood supply—the pulp—so diabetes causes a reduction in blood flow to the pulp, which lowers the tooth's immune defense system. This is one of the reasons why diabetics have so many tooth issues; they simply cannot heal.

The majority of people will never get checked for diabetes. The danger in that is that people with insulin resistance (prediabetes) can be asymptomatic for up to ten years. It is estimated that 10.8 percent of adults have prediabetes, 11.3 percent have diabetes, and 22.7 percent have diabetes *but are undiagnosed.*[19] Or in other words, approximately one-half of American adults have either insulin resistance issues or full-onset diabetes. Unfortunately, the problem of diabetes isn't restricted to blood vessels. When left untreated, it can become the starting point for other diseases, such as kidney disease, dementia, retinopathy, heart disease, neuropathy, and periodontal disease, to have complications—a "gateway disease," if you will.

With so many people falling victim to diabetes, it only makes sense to look into the reasons why.

THE CAUSE

Diabetes occurs in two ways: type 1 and type 2 (real creative, I know). Type 1 is often referred to as juvenile diabetes (though it doesn't *have* to come to fruition during childhood, and frankly, more and more people are being diagnosed with it as adults).

---

19 Centers for Disease Control and Prevention, "National Diabetes Statistic Report: Estimates of Diabetes and Its Burden in the United States," last reviewed June 29, 2022, https://www.cdc.gov/diabetes/data/statistics-report/index.html.

It is generally understood to be an autoimmune disorder. It is not preventable and occurs with bad luck. While there are cases where adults contract a virus that attacks the pancreas and causes type 1 diabetes, that is uncommon. No one is completely sure why the body develops this condition.

In type 1, the body attacks and kills the pancreas cells (beta islet cells) responsible for making insulin, halting its production. The result is that the patient needs an external source of insulin for the rest of their lives, usually provided through an insulin pump.

A brief explanation of insulin: insulin is the hormone responsible for controlling the uptake of sugar from our blood into cells. This is how our cells get the energy they need to operate. With diabetes, no insulin means no uptake of sugar from the bloodstream into the cells to be used for energy, and that means cellular functions cannot be performed. The cells get no energy. Without intervention, type 1 diabetics would die at an early age.

Type 2 diabetes has the same dysfunctions as type 1, but this version of the disease is often attributed to lifestyle and diet and is *mostly* preventable. Type 2 comprises 90 percent of all diabetes cases. The difference between types 1 and 2 is that in type 1, the body attacks and destroys the insulin-producing cells. In type 2, the body cannot make enough insulin to keep up with demand or the insulin does not work properly. Type 1: no insulin. Type 2: ineffective/insufficient insulin. We will focus on type 2 for this chapter.

THE MOUTH-VASCULAR CONNECTION (TYPE 2 DIABETES)

In the medical world, we're still unsure if diabetes causes periodontal disease, and vice versa, or if there's any causal connection at all, but the numbers show that the correlation is evident regardless. Bidirectional or not, one ailment clearly increases the risk and severity of the other. One connection is the same as with the heart; it all goes back to Chapter 2 and the leaky gum problem I described (you'll see a running theme here).

The manifested issue depends on the particular bacteria that happens to penetrate your bloodstream. In the case of diabetes, the main offenders are Aa, Td, Tf, Pg, and Fn (you'll see there is lots of overlap among the bacteria related to heart disease). These five bacteria are thought to be the most responsible for causing chronic inflammation that could lead to damage of the pancreas's ability to create and secrete insulin. In this scenario, poor oral health can lead to diabetes.

However, the reverse can also be true: high blood sugar can cause oral health problems. There are a few different factors at play with that, one of which is saliva.

SPIT TAKE

Saliva production is crucial to overall wellness. For starters, it secretes an enzyme called amylase that predigests food (it does a particularly good job of breaking down carbohydrates). Saliva lubricates the mouth, which aids in swallowing and prevents choking. It also protects us from cavities by coating and remineralizing our teeth, and—on a fun note—it helps us taste our food!

Let's back up to that coating and remineralizing our teeth thing… Our saliva creates a natural biofilm called a pellicle—a thin protective layer made up of good bacteria and proteins on our teeth—that delays an invasive form of a harmful biofilm. A lack of saliva makes your teeth more "sticky," which causes bad bacteria to collect quickly. Those bacteria eat away at the mineral exterior of your teeth, beginning the decay process. Xerostomia (dry mouth) is something that diabetic patients often suffer from because the chronic inflammation associated with diabetes decreases the sublingual and parotid glands' (the spit-making bits) ability to produce saliva. Their frequent dry mouth, then, provides bacteria with ample time to eat away at teeth.

Remember: when we are chronically stressed and in fight-or-flight mode, our digestive system shuts down. Who wants to poop when you're running from a tiger? Unfortunately, saliva production is a part of our digestive system. So individuals who are chronically stressed suffer from dry mouth and more tooth issues.

Stay with me here...those bacteria piling up on the sticky teeth don't just sit there. More is happening inside the diabetic's mouth that enables the bacteria to destroy teeth by creating cavities. That enabler is sugar.

IT'S STILL ABOUT THE SUGAR

Cavities are often caused by the *Strep. mutans* bacteria, which thrive off of sugars, especially processed sugars like the ones found in bread and sodas, key foods that can lead to type 2 diabetes. Making things worse, what saliva a diabetic does have is *jam-packed* with sugar (just like with the sugar in their blood). All that sugar provides a feeding ground for bad bacteria. It eats it up and poops out acid (you're not hard-core unless you live hard-core), which eats away at your tooth enamel. So basically, a cavity is a microscopic latrine of corrosive excrement.

But that's not all! You know what else loves sugar? *Fungus.* With all the immune system has to constantly fend off, other infections start to insert themselves in your body, most notably fungal. Diabetics will also often have pale and cracked tongues (thrush) and develop angular cheilitis (cracked and crusty corners of the mouth/lips), both of which are due to fungal overgrowth.

An interesting side effect of diabetes (especially type 1) is that the sugar in the saliva causes a patient's breath to smell sweet or like alcohol.

PERPETUAL ILLNESS, MORE TROUBLE, AND HOPE

So by now, you can see the connection between poor oral health possibly causing diabetes and diabetes making it harder to have good oral health. It might be a chicken-and-egg matter, or it could be a both/and matter. Regardless, it's important to recognize the connection. Studies show that periodontal disease increases your risk for type 2 diabetes by 50 to 100 percent; meanwhile, A1C levels are higher in diabetic patients with periodontal disease versus those without.[20] In other words, periodontal disease makes diabetes worse, and vice versa.

Think of the relationship between diabetes and periodontal disease as a perpetual dance of death. Diabetes hampers the body's healing and bacteria-fighting abilities, making mouth infections all the more severe, which is why diabetics are more prone to tooth and gum abscesses. And the chronic oral inflam-

---

20 David A. Albert et al., "Diabetes and Oral Disease: Implications for Health Professionals," *Annals of the New York Academy of Sciences* 1255, no. 1 Annals *Meeting Reports* (March 2012): 1–15, https://doi.org/10.1111/j.1749-6632.2011.06460.x.

mation and infection that occur with periodontal disease grow and spread throughout the body via MMP-8. This exacerbates systemic inflammation…which magnifies the mouth condition…which spreads to the body…now spin, now chassé…The dance goes on.

As bad as it is already, the nightmare cocktail of diabetes and periodontal disease gets worse; one way is by dysregulating bone formation. Normally, our bodies are in a balanced state of bone degradation and formation (we remake our bones much like how a snake sheds its skin). Osteoporosis is the upset of this balance due to a change in hormones, like after menopause: the body builds less bone than it breaks down. Diabetes-aggravated periodontal disease essentially creates the same imbalance in the mouth by permanently activating osteoclasts (the bone tearer-downers). The osteoblasts (the bone builder-uppers) can't keep up, and the bones degrade. This is why patients with uncontrolled diabetes lose an enormous amount of bone in their teeth, so much so that sometimes their teeth fall out on their own.

And last but not least, there is strong evidence that shows periodontal disease increases the risk of end-stage diabetes complications like cardiovascular disease and kidney disease.

But it's not all bad news.

YOUR DENTIST CAN HELP!

Your dentist can be the first person to recognize signs that you may be prediabetic or even diabetic. I can usually spot diabetes the moment someone gets into my chair. Typically, in the early stages, I'll see red and swollen bleeding gums that don't quite correlate to the amount of bone loss present in their mouths; in early stages, diabetes presents itself more as acute inflammation rather than full-on gum disease (a case of chronic inflammation would have had more time to break down the teeth). Obviously, bone degradation will occur down the road if the diabetes is left untreated, but inflamed gums and cavities are the immediate giveaways, especially around the gingival margin (the portion of gum tissue that's directly around the neck of the tooth). The reason is that the gingival margin is where the would-be protective biofilm settles, and since diabetics have xerostomia, this protective pellicle is missing. Their tissues will feel sticky because they are dry and will be pale pink in color.

After you receive a diagnosis of diabetes and/or periodontal disease, your dentist will recommend that you stay on a strict ninety-day cleaning cycle. This is because periodontal cleanings are shown to provide a 0.4 percent drop in A1C levels (every 1 percent drop in A1C is related to a 14 to 21 percent drop in end-stage diabetic symptoms).[21] However, bad bacteria repopulate, and this benefit only lasts around ninety days at a time, which is why your dentist wants to schedule a cleaning around every three months. (*See?* Dentists aren't just after your wallet.) The goal of these frequent cleanings is to minimize bad bacterial numbers and inflammation and prevent the bacteria from entering your bloodstream and feeding diabetes.

If you have diabetes, you should include oral healthcare in your disease management plan—simple, nonsurgical perio treatment, along with regular maintenance and brushing and flossing are effective and affordable means to help you significantly reduce your inflammation. There is an old joke in dentistry: only floss the teeth you intend to keep!

---

21   Albert et al., "Diabetes and Oral Disease."

Imagine if Sue had known all of this when she experienced her first diabetic symptoms. How would her life have turned out? How much suffering could she have been spared? Even in her old age, she decided to try a risky procedure just to get some relief. Fortunately, the science (and luck) held up; her body accepted the operation, and she lives a much better life now. I am writing this book for that reason; I don't want anyone to suffer for lack of knowledge. I want to share these truths so people can act on them ASAP.

Next, we'll discuss how oral health connects to the life-altering diagnosis that so many unfortunate people are given every day.

Cancer.

CHAPTER 5

The C-Word

WE'RE GOING TO TALK ABOUT CANCER AND HOW YOUR dentist can save your life. And no, that isn't hyperbole. Listen up.

I had a new patient, named Linda, who came into my office for an initial exam. While reviewing her medical history, I saw she had had cervical cancer several years earlier. Luckily, it had been detected in its early stages, and with surgery and treatment, she told me, it resolved quickly with no recurrence. Other than that, she was fit as a fiddle.

When I start my checkups, I like to do a quick scan with the naked eye—to the trained professional, many oral issues stand out as obvious. Everything looked great on the surface; she had a healthy mouth and a healthy set of gums. However, no matter what, we always use an oral abnormality detection device called a VELscope™ on our patients.

A VELscope is a painless "flashlight" that allows us to see the cellular activity beneath our surface tissue that indicates something is amiss, such as pathology/cancer, trauma, and/or infection. Think of it like looking under the hood of a car—the surface could be waxed and polished, but the engine may be a mess. The idea behind this tool is that it detects the increased DNA activity that occurs in infection, inflammation, trauma, or even cancer. When any of those things happen, DNA begins replicating for healing purposes, cells morph into cancerous ones, and/or bacteria start having a field day (all examples of "increased DNA activity"). Because these more cellularly active areas are denser, they don't let the light from the VELscope through; they appear darker than their surroundings, revealing their presence beneath the surface. It's kind of like those children's books where you shine a light behind the page to see a tiger hiding in the grass or a secret message. The entire process only takes a minute or two and is highly recommended, as the nature of oral abnormalities makes them easily hidden in the anatomy and difficult to detect (more on that later).

When I used the VELscope on Linda, it revealed a lesion on her right tonsil—something invisible with my initial look-see. Knowing there was a link between cervical cancer and oropharyngeal cancer, we immediately sent her for a biopsy. The report came back as stage 0 cancer linked to HPV (human papillomavirus). Yes, stage 0. That means the cancer had *just* started and hadn't had the chance to even spread within the tissue where it originated. Catching cancer like this is as close as doctors come to being clairvoyant.

Because the cancer was caught so early, Linda was successfully treated by removing her tonsils (a tonsillectomy). Once again Linda had no recurrence. As icing on the cake, she neither lost her sense of taste nor suffered xerostomia (that's dry mouth for the memory impaired), all because the early discovery allowed for minimal treatment.

While Linda's story is proof positive that your dentist's screening for oral cancer is important, there is also—surprise!—a connection between the bacteria in your mouth and cancers found elsewhere in your body. In other words, the mouth-cancer connection is multifaceted. Let's first take it from the top and begin our cancer discussion with our mouths, with oral cancer, and then we'll get into the nitty-gritty of bacteria and how it might be contributing to pancreatic and colon cancers.

IT'S (NOT) CANCER SEASON

Let's first start out by talking about what cancer is. In short, cancer is when a cell goes rogue. When cells divide, as they tend to do to keep us alive and everything in good working order, they are supposed to replicate themselves exactly. That's what DNA and RNA and probably a few other NAs are all about: the coding necessary for a cell to be godlike and remake itself in its own image. When it doesn't do that and instead makes a slightly different cell, that cell can't function like it's supposed to. And then when it replicates its misfit self, it starts a whole gang of cells that don't function in a way that becomes optimal. If left to their own devices long enough, those cells will create a tumor or show up as a patch of melanoma on a person's cheek. In addition, when normal cells screw up this process and don't make perfect replicas, their inbuilt safety mechanism switches on and they self-destruct (so they don't grow into something worse). With cancer cells, however, this "suicide button" is permanently turned off, allowing the misfits to keep on keepin' on.

So if you're thinking the best way to prevent cancer is by preventing cells from going bad, pat yourself on the back. You're absolutely right. So then the next question is: Why does that happen to begin with? Why do they have identity crises and create alternate selves?

You already know the answer to that question. It's what Chapter 2 was all about: inflammation.

Chronic inflammation has been linked to just about every stage of cancer. In layman's terms, inflammation aids cancer cells by helping them create their own blood supply, allowing them to replicate and live longer. It can shut down healthy cells and make it easier for cancer cells to spread throughout the body.[22] Cancer also thrives in inflamed tissues.

In other words: stop inflammation, and you can stop the development of most (possibly all) cancers.

How do you stop inflammation? You know one of the answers already: good oral health!

Additionally, do all those things your doctor has been telling you to do for years: eat a healthy diet, don't gain too much weight, don't smoke, sleep more, and on and on and on. You get the picture. Now let's look at what we need to talk about for this book, beginning with oral cancer.

ORAL CANCER AND WHY IT SUCKS

Consider oral cancer (OC) to be any cancer in the oral cavity—lips, tongue, the floor of the mouth, gums, tonsils, and oropharynx (the part of the throat at the back of the mouth) included. Oral cancer is particularly nasty as it is often only discovered in its later stages after it has metastasized and spread down into the lymphatic/circulatory system (that's *real* bad, FYI). The reason is that oral cancer starts growing in areas that are undetectable and beneath the surface (a dentist glancing in your mouth with their overhead light won't do). Hence, me harping on the VELscope. OC starts beneath the surface. If the Velscope does detect something abnormal, the patient will be

---

22 Nitin Singh et al., "Inflammation and Cancer," *Annals of African Medicine* 18, no. 3 (2019): 121–126, https://doi.org/10.4103/aam.aam_56_18.

sent for a biopsy to obtain a clinical diagnosis. The Velscope detects abnormalities; it does not diagnose cancer.

It's often discovered so late because most forms of mouth cancer have a reddish color, which, in addition to the anatomical structure of the mouth, makes oral cancer somewhat camouflaged and difficult to detect. OC can vary in appearance depending on its location and can range from a nonhealing ulcer (especially on the lips) to lumps under the skin. With tongue cancer, tumors most often occur on the sides of the tongue; floor-of-the-mouth cancer has the same side action going on.

With cheek cancer, red and white velvety lesions form at the base of the cheeks, which, strangely enough, is just about the same spot where people hold their chewing tobacco (sarcasm *heavily* implied). Cancer in the back of the throat tends to be asymmetrical and blends in with anatomy. (I mean, just look at your tonsils. They already look like they don't belong.)

At times, these manifestations can appear white, giving them contrast to our red mouths and making them more readily detectable. Or patients will feel a lump as they swallow or find a swollen lymph node in their neck or under their chin, which is a dead giveaway, pun intended. (Note: lumps lasting less than two weeks are generally considered safe.) In other occurrences, patients' voices will suddenly become hoarse. If these earlier signs can be detected, your dentist can perform a more thorough scan with an oral abnormality tool, such as ViziLite, Bio/Screen, OralID, or my favorite, *VELscope* (okay, okay, I won't mention it anymore). Of course, it is always advised to go see your regular doctor right away as they can do advanced imaging to detect and diagnose the actual lesion, because we're dentists, after all, not doctors—at least not doctors who specialize in diagnosing lesions.

Oral cancer ranks as the twelfth-most common cancer in the US and as the sixteenth-most deadly. It affects twice as many men as women and is more prevalent in white people and those who are overweight, especially those who eat crappy foods, like processed meats and sugar. And with vaping and HPV diagnoses on the rise, I predict the incidence of OC will rise as well.

WHERE DOES IT COME FROM?

Right, inflammation. Smoking doesn't just cause lung cancer. Lip cancers form due to cigarette heat causing a burn injury, leading to cellular damage (lips burn easily, and burns are inflammation). Cancers of the tongue and floor of the mouth are also typically caused by tobacco use (smoking or chewing nicotine causes inflammation) as well as by excessive alcohol consumption (another inflammatory habit—are you seeing a pattern here?).[23] In fact, for smokers who are also excessive alcohol drinkers, their risk of developing oral cancer is *thirty times higher*. Last but not least, cigarettes are full of toxic, cancer-causing chemicals that *never* would be allowed to be ingested on their own, but somehow (maybe something to do with billions of dollars) they're okay when you smoke them together; *got a light?*

Interestingly, despite the number of smokers decreasing over the years, the amount of oral cancers is rising slightly. That's due to the HPV virus, which is responsible for 50 percent of all throat cancer and 30 percent of all oral cancer. It is also the virus responsible for cervical/anal cancers, certain warts, and

---

23 Umea University, "One More Reason to Swear Off Tobacco: The Inflammatory Trap Induced by Nicotine," *Science Daily*, news release, September 1, 2016, www.sciencedaily.com/releases/2016/09/160901124842.htm; H. Joe Wang, Samir Zakhari, and M. Katherine Jung, "Alcohol, Inflammation, and Gut-Liver-Brain Interactions in Tissue Damage and Disease Development," *World Journal of Gastroenterology* 16, no. 11 (2010): 1304–1313, https://doi.org/10.3748/wjg.v16.i11.1304.

abnormal Pap smears. It is highly advised that if you've ever had an abnormal Pap smear or cervical cancer, you get an oral cancer screening.

Almost all adults will contract HPV at some point in their lives, but the majority of the infections will resolve on their own (unbeknownst to the host). Smoking comes into play here, because people exposed to tobacco smoke are less likely to clear the infection from their bodies.[24] HPV is also transmitted sexually—*you fill in the blanks*—which might explain why one in five cases of OC is now in people younger than fifty-five.[25]

STATING THE OBVIOUS

You may have noticed that the causes of OC mostly come from lifestyle habits. That's right: oral cancer is almost *entirely* preventable. As you can see in the following chart, two of the most common vices in this country—smokin' 'n' drinkin'—are associated with 68 percent of tongue cancers and 52 percent of cancers on the floor of the mouth (FOM).

CANCER LOCATION	FREQUENCY	CAUSE
Tongue	68%	Tobacco, Drinking
FOM	52%	Tobacco, Drinking
Oropharynx	50%	HPV

---

24 Carole Fakhry, Maura L. Gillison, and Gypsyamber D'Souza, "Tobacco Use and Oral HPV-16 Infection," *JAMA* 312, no. 14 (2014): 1465–1467, https://doi.org/10.1001/jama.2014.13183.

25 American Cancer Society, "Key Statistics for Oral Cavity and Oropharyngeal Cancers," last revised January 18, 2023, https://www.cancer.org/cancer/oral-cavity-and-oropharyngeal-cancer/about/key-statistics.html.

Practicing safe sex and living a healthy lifestyle free from smoking and drinking will dramatically reduce the odds of you developing oral cancer.

To be fair, there are a few genetic mutations that contribute to oral cancer risk. But being that these are so few and far between, I regularly only preach on the preventable nature of OC to my patients. Let's control what we can control.

A LITTLE GOOD NEWS

On a positive note, HPV-related oral cancer has been shown to be quite responsive to chemotherapy and radiation treatments, which creates better outcomes and greatly lifts the survival rate. And, in general, survival rates of all oral cancers are on the rise! This is largely due to the development of technology that is better and faster at detecting OC, having more effective treatments available, and the overall number of smokers decreasing. Though, due to OC still typically only being discovered in its later stages, the quality of life after a resolution is grim. Surviving patients are often left deformed (including missing parts of their jaw, lips, and/or tongue) and experience painful mouth sores, a burning tongue, and/or a lack of taste. The moral of the story here is just because you *can* survive oral cancer doesn't mean you shouldn't take it seriously.

Last Dance with What's-Her-Face (Mary Jane)

It's important that I add a note about marijuana here. For whatever reason, marijuana has become associated with cancer treatment. Let me be clear: THC *does* have positive effects on anxiety and pain relief, inducing sleep, and stimulating the appetite that helps cancer and AIDS patients gain weight.

But the hubbub on the subject is that THC has cancer-killing effects—*no such claim has been substantiated by strong evidence.* And for all the evidence that shows THC *fights* cancer, there is just as much that shows it *causes* cancer. Regardless, many of the benefits of THC come with side effects that are counterproductive when concerning oral cancer. For example, while marijuana does help thin people gain body mass by giving them "the munchies," there's a reason there's a late-night food truck franchise called Insomniac Cookies and not Insomniac Fruits and Veggies. The appetite stimulus caused by THC generally drives people toward unhealthy foods that increase decay and inflammation.

For marijuana smokers, in particular, the problem gets worse. The smoke generated by smoking THC is quite toxic, containing many of the same by-products as cigarette smoke ("But it's like…from the earth, man…"). Cannabis stomatitis is quite common amongst heavy marijuana smokers, and, if you're unaware, includes gingival enlargement (gum expansion), chronic oral inflammation (leading to leaky gums), and leukoplakia (white, hairy patches of tissue in the mouth). Yeah…try and convince me that blazin' a doob is healthy when you've got hair growing on your tongue. (But if you insist on smoking all those left-handed cigarettes, you might bring back the days of having a barber take care of oral care too.) Back to the point, with cannabis stomatitis comes what naturally would with any stomatitis: bone loss, periodontal disease, and comparatively more cavities (as opposed to someone who doesn't smoke weed).

THC has also recently been discovered to be immunosuppressive. Meaning if a marijuana user has an HPV infection, they will have an increased risk of it developing into head and neck cancer. The reason is that THC, while decreasing cell death (apoptosis) in some cancers, actually allows HPV cancer cells to grow uncontrollably.[26]

And last but not least, it's widely known that marijuana causes "cotton mouth," which is just another way of saying xerostomia. This, as discussed in the previous chapter, gives bad bacteria everything they need to wreak havoc on your mouth. Whether it's a vape, tobacco, or the devil's lettuce, the heat caused by smoking constricts the blood vessels in your mouth, and this restriction of blood flow is what lessens your immune response.

What I'm not saying is "weed is bad"—the evidence is inconclusive at best. What I'm trying to do is address all those who view smoking and vaping THC as a healthy alternative to cigarettes. There's more to this issue that the public needs to be made aware of.

* * *

Hopefully, you can see by now why your dentist wants to do a cancer screening every time you go in for a cleaning. With tools such as the VELscope, we are in a prime spot to find oral cancers early in their progression. But the mouth-cancer connection doesn't stop there. As we've seen in heart disease and diabetes, bacteria in the mouth can impact cancer elsewhere in the body. In this case, Aa, Pg, Td, Tf, and Fn have been connected to pancreas, colon, esophageal, lung, and head and neck cancers. I'll go over a specific few now that we can say for sure have a connection to oral bacteria.

---

26 Yadira Galindo, "How Marijuana Accelerates Growth of HPV-Related Head and Neck Cancer Identified," UC San Diego Health, news release, January 13, 2020, https://health.ucsd.edu/news/releases/Pages/2020-01-13-how-marijuana-accelerates-growth-of-hpv-related-head-and-neck-cancer-identified.aspx.

PANCREATIC CANCER

Pancreatic cancer (PC) is a bad one. Because the pancreas is located behind major organs, it often creates pain elsewhere in the body when damaged, and when there is a problem with it, there is a relative lack of symptoms (at most, a gallbladder issue). Therefore, PC is difficult to detect and, because of this, is typically only found in stage 4 (a later stage).[27] Also, due to its location, the pancreas is nearly impossible to isolate and treat with chemotherapy or radiation. Although pancreatic cancer is uncommon, because of these complications, the five-year survival rate can be as low as 3 percent, making it the third-leading cause of cancer deaths. So it's a high priority for us to be aware of the warning signs.[28] One of which is oral health.

Periodontal disease is associated with a 59 percent increased risk of PC, and it's currently being unveiled that PC is also associated with high levels of Pg in the saliva. In truth, pancreatic cancer is connected to high levels of Aa and Pg, but it's Pg that's the real culprit, as people are 67 percent more likely to develop pancreatic cancer with a Pg infection. Several studies are now looking at the link between oral bacteria and pancreatic cancer more closely, and the University of California San Diego is refining a saliva test that will check for specific enzymes and Pg in saliva, all in an effort to start catching PC earlier.[29]

27 Dominique S. Michaud et al., "A Prospective Study of Periodontal Disease and Pancreatic Cancer in US Male Health Professionals," *Journal of the National Cancer Institute* 99, no. 2 (January 2007): 171–175, https://doi.org/10.1093/jnci/djk021; Pancreatic Cancer Action Network, "Pancreatic Cancer Facts 2016," February 2016, https://www.pancan.org/wp-content/uploads/2016/02/2016-GAA-PC-Facts.pdf.

28 Cancer.Net, "Pancreatic Cancer: Statistics," February 2022, https://www.cancer.net/cancer-types/pancreatic-cancer/statistics.

29 "Bacteria in Mouth May Diagnose Pancreatic Cancer," Science Daily, May 18, 2014, https://www.sciencedaily.com/releases/2014/05/140518164419.htm.

Colon cancer is the development of cancerous lesions (or polyps) in the colon, which are easily detectable via a colonoscopy or at-home test such as Cologuard. While most polyps are benign, they can turn cancerous. So it is common practice to remove all polyps to be safe, just as it is with some moles. The five-year survival rate for colon cancer is 64 percent. However, if found during its localized stage, the rate jumps up to 91 percent. You can see why regular checkups for those over fifty years old are encouraged.

So the question then, is why do the polyps form? The answer, at least partially, lies in *Fusobacterium nucleatum*. (It's the Fn bacterium, if you've forgotten.) Guess what bacterium causes 20 percent of all colon cancer. Yep, Fn. Maybe you'd never place a bet on 20 percent odds. However, Fn does more than just cause those cancers within; it increases the chances for colon cancer recurrence and makes it harder for chemo treatments to beat cancer.[30] Here's how Fn commits its crimes.

Fn colonizes in the intestines, and from there it works its way down to the colon and placenta (hence the gestational complications of Fn infection, but we'll discuss that in a later chapter). To build their colonies, the bacteria stick to the lining of the colon, which increases the permeability of the intestines, creating leaky gut syndrome (as I'll discuss in the next chapter) and inciting inflammation.

When you have bad bacteria in the gut, it creates a microbiome dysbiosis (disruption), which raises the risk of colon

---

30   Chun-Hui Sun et al., "The Role of *Fusobacterium nucleatum* in Colorectal Cancer: From Carcinogenesis to Clinical Management," *Chronic Diseases and Translational Medicine* 5, no. 3 (2019): 178–187, https://doi.org/10.1016/j.cdtm.2019.09.001; Jiao Wu, Qing Li, and Xiangsheng Fu, "*Fusobacterium nucleatum* Contributes to the Carcinogenesis of Colorectal Cancer by Inducing Inflammation and Suppressing Host Immunity," *Translational Oncology* 12, no. 6 (June 2019): 846–851, https://doi.org/10.1016/j.tranon.2019.03.003.

cancer *and* increases its carcinogenicity by the differentiation and proliferation of epithelial cells. Put more simply, when the cells lining your colon are disrupted by bad bacteria, they have trouble cloning themselves to make new healthy cells. Instead, they become mutated, and mutated cells are where the origins of cancer can be found. When those mutated cells reproduce themselves enough times, they create cancerous polyps and tumors.

In addition, it's been discovered that when Fn is present in the colon, colonic tumors will have four times the amount of Fn than the surrounding tissue—Fn seems to be drawn to polyps.[31]

Okay, but What about the Mouth?

If you've been following along closely, you will have noticed that I haven't mentioned how the mouth ties into colon cancer. Let's address that. Beyond the fact that Fn is present in the mouth, colon cancer patients have also been shown to have abnormally high levels of Pg in their mouths. Oral Pg is well known to invade the gut and promote tumor progression. So basically, an oral infection of Pg paves the way for Fn to cause colon cancer, thus connecting periodontal disease to colon cancer. Plus, studies have shown that oral Fn, intestinal Fn, and high plaque/gingival index scores are all correlated to colon cancer.[32]

---

31   Jii Bum Lee et al., "Association between *Fusobacterium nucleatum* and Patient Prognosis in Metastatic Colon Cancer," *Scientific Reports* 11 (2021), https://doi.org/10.1038/s41598-021-98941-6.

32   Harvard T. H. Chan School of Public Health, "Gum Disease Associated with Higher Gastrointestinal, Colon Cancer Risk," news release, July 31, 2020, https://www.hsph.harvard.edu/news/hsph-in-the-news/gum-disease-gastrointestinal-cancer-risk.

Treatment

One of the worst things about Fn-induced colon cancer is that Fn is more resistant to chemotherapy, and since Fn likes to pack itself into colon tumors, colon cancer is more resistant to chemotherapy in turn. Fn is also associated with colon cancer recurrence. So instead of the typical cancer treatments, an antibiotic designed to specifically kill Fn, called metronidazole, is used as one treatment modality for Fn-associated colon cancers (all of which would be prescribed by your doctor).[33] Oh, and a plus for all you vegetarians: higher levels of intestinal Fn are associated with eating red meat. Sorry, Atkins fans.

THE MOUTH-CANCER CONNECTION

If nothing else, recognize that even cancer is connected to oral health and that your dentist has the ability to detect the oral bacteria that are known to correlate with certain cancers as well as to help you keep your mouth healthy to prevent unnecessary inflammation. But on top of that, your dentist can find those elusive mouth cancers *extremely* early. Think of where Linda would be right now if she were one of those who "only go to the dentist when they have a problem." Schedule an exam and start seeing your dentist on the regular. They might just save your life.

For example, I had a long-term patient whose teeth I was quite familiar with, and for all the years I'd known her she'd been healthy. However, one day she came in for her regular checkup and just looked *bad*. I suspected something was wrong, and once I got her in the chair, I knew it for sure.

Her gums were bleeding, and she had *tons* of plaque. I asked

---

33 Jing-yuan Fang, "Study of Oral Metronidazole on Postoperative Chemotherapy in Colorectal Cancer," clinical trial, ClinicalTrials.gov identifier NCT04264676, last updated November 25, 2020, https://clinicaltrials.gov/ct2/show/NCT04264676.

if anything was wrong, and it turned out she'd just been diagnosed with stage 2 rectal cancer. So I ran an oral DNA test, and wouldn't you know it? She had an Fn infection. I immediately contacted her doctor, and we put her on metronidazole. I asked her why she hadn't come to see me earlier, and she said, "Well, doc. Because it's in my ass, and you're a dentist." It was certainly understandable, but believe me, I lectured her on the mouth-body connection.

While it's possible the oral infection contributed to her cancer, we don't know for sure. Other culprits (like diet) could have been at play. But why risk it? If perio treatments can curtail cancer risk, why not get the freaking treatments? Whether my patient's gum disease led to her cancer or not, inflammation is nothing to ignore. In fact, inflammation can be a disease in and of itself. This is what we'll focus on next, specifically on inflammatory diseases like arthritis and bowel disease. But first, we'll start with the telltale sign of how healthy your insides are: your poop.

CHAPTER 6

Inflammation and Poop: When Things Get Messy

AS A DENTIST, I HAVE THE WONDERFUL PRIVILEGE OF treating family members (it comes with the territory, as with most professions). One of my family members is *obsessed* with health. She's young (in her early thirties) and does "all the things": strictly eats an unprocessed and organic-only diet, takes supplements, is religious about her sleep schedule, hits the gym at 5:00 a.m. five to six days a week, only drinks on occasion, and *never* smokes. She's the picture of health, to say the least, and I'd be lying if I didn't say I wasn't a little jealous.

Largely due to her regimen, she's also never had a cavity. In fact, other dentists have told her that she flosses *too* much (blasphemy!). Now, I did say she is obsessed with her health; remember that as I tell you this next part. Something she prides herself on is her healthy poop—she examines it every day. If you didn't throw up in your mouth just now, let me tell you why that is actually one of the best things she can do (and you too).

Because she (you know why I left her unnamed now) was

so familiar with her poop, not long ago, she noticed when the shape of her poop and frequency of bowel movements changed. In addition, she didn't feel "empty" after pooping and started feeling inflamed and swollen. The rest of our family blew her off because she was so healthy and, like I said, she is a bit over the top with all this. Despite that, she had a physical and blood work done on herself. Strangely (but not surprisingly), they both came back as normal.

Soon thereafter, she came into my office for the routine checkup—hers were *very* routine and typically took less than thirty minutes because of her supreme health. However, this time was different…Her gums were bleeding like a stuck pig! Obviously, this was not the norm for her and had to be serious, so I immediately took X-rays. The X-rays showed the beginnings of mild bone loss (a huge change from six months prior). I remembered her complaining about her gut/poop issues, so I also ran an MMP-8 test, and the results were astonishing. On the MMP-8 test, any result over sixty is considered severe systemic inflammation and collagen breakdown (leaky gut)—her results were at *eighty-three*! We were both shocked, as six months before this, her results were below a healthy twenty.

I delivered nonsurgical periodontal therapy (deep cleaning, microbial irrigants, localized antibiotics, lasers) and suggested a few supplements to add to her regimen. She saw an immediate improvement in her poop. (She also went to a gastroenterologist the next day for a previously scheduled appointment who said everything was fine from his end. Go figure!)

Update: her poop improved for a few weeks but regressed again. I saw her for a follow-up cleaning three months later, and her MMP improved to forty-three, but her gums were still messy. She saw a functional medicine doctor who diagnosed her with SIBO (small intestine bacterial overgrowth). Although we were able to improve her gums a little, something was still off, so the SIBO diagnosis made sense. We cannot get full health unless the microbiomes in both the mouth *and* the gut are healthy.

As I've been saying, the body is systemic; everything is connected, and now you know I mean *everything*. My family member was aware of this fact and used her poop to discover a problem *in her mouth*. Poop is like a litmus test for inflammation in the body, and inflammation causes a myriad of ailments. However, inflammation itself can be a problem, especially with issues like bowel disease and arthritis. Let's dive in and connect all the dots.

AN INTRODUCTION TO POOP AND THE GUT

The US loves poop—or, at least, we love the gut. Gut health has almost reached fad status in America. Because our poop can tell us just how our gut is feeling, many influencers, products, clinics, and medical/wellness practices have dedicated themselves to poop health.

Analyzing poop is like digging through someone's trash—it tells you a lot about a person. Poop can reveal if someone has a fungal infection (white slime on the poop), viral/bacterial infection (stringy, watery, nonfunctional poop), cancer (bloody stool can imply colon cancer, later confirmed with a fecal lab test), or gut dysbiosis (diarrhea or constipation is a sign of there being more bad bacteria than good).

Poop shows us what foods our bodies like and do not like. (Think about the last burrito that "disagreed" with you. Who won that argument? Not your pants, I'm guessing.) Poop even gives clues about your hormone levels (progesterone is associated with constipation—*as if pregnant women needed any more issues to deal with*). It all comes down to our gut microbiome;

the biome's health determines the poop's health. Our gut micro-biome is considered our "second brain."

The human body actually has ten times more microbial cells than, well, human cells. Right: we're made up of a bunch of bacteria! A study on the genetic material in the microbiome found that there are 3.3 million unique genes in the human gut—that's 150 times more genes than our human genome has. Those genes make up the nearly 1,000 different bacterial species living inside us. But they're not freeloaders. Our gut bacteria are critical for regulating gut metabolism and a strong immune system.[34]

The idea does hold some truth; 90 percent of serotonin (the feel-good hormone) is created by the cells that line the digestive tract, which is the reason why depression, anxiety, and mood disorders are connected to inflammatory bowel disease.[35] When the lining of the intestines is damaged—you know, inflamed—serotonin production is disrupted, and sufferers wind up with both mental *and* digestive issues. Ensure that your gut (and emotions) stay healthy by consuming good-gut-bacteria-promoting fermented foods such as kombucha, kefir, and pre/probiotics, as well as fiber. Neurotransmitters are made up of amino acids, so make sure to get enough protein!

---

34 Baoli Zhu, Xin Wang, and Lanjuan Li, "Human Gut Microbiome: The Second Genome of Human Body," *Protein & Cell* 1, no. 8 (August 2010): 718–725, https://doi.org/10.1007/s13238-010-0093-z.

35 G. B. Rogers et al., "From Gut Dysbiosis to Altered Brain Function and Mental Illness: Mechanisms and Pathways," *Molecular Psychology* 21 (2016): 738–748, https://doi.org/10.1038/mp.2016.50; N. A. Koloski, M. Jones, and N. J. Talley, "Evidence That Independent Gut-to-Brain and Brain-to-Gut Pathways Operate in the Irritable Bowel Syndrome and Functional Dyspepsia: A 1-Year Population-Based Prospective Study," *Alimentary Pharmacology & Therapeutics* 44, no. 6 (September 2016): 592–600, https://doi.org/10.1111/apt.13738.

The gut is the largest bacterial microbiome in the body, home to more than 100 trillion bacteria. And what starts it off? The mouth! The implication is obvious; our mouth's microbiome (the second largest in the body) completely determines the state of our gut's microbiome (because we swallow it). Speaking on the oral microbiome isn't as sexy as speaking on gut health—not yet, at least (I'm starting a new fad). But the truth is that there are more than 700 million bacteria in our mouths, encompassing 700 different species. Needless to say, we need to nurture our oral microbiome. It affects everything else. And it's where dysbiosis in the body can start.

THE MOUTH-BOWEL DISEASE CONNECTION

I'm not really saying anything profound; your mouth is the beginning of your digestive system, and what goes in from the top winds up in your gut. If you are still a little suspicious (most people are), just look up Crohn's disease and the mouth. Crohn's disease, an inflammatory bowel disease, has well-documented symptoms of a "cobblestone appearance" in the gums.

Whenever I see this at my practice, I ask, "Hey, having some gut issues?" Every time, I get "Yeah, how'd you know?" in response. I know because it's all the same systemic problem; there's inflammation in the gut, and it's manifesting in the gums. It's all the same tissue. Researchers have found increased numbers of oral bacteria in the intestines of people with bowel diseases.[36]

---

36 Koji Atarashi et al., "Ectopic Colonization of Oral Bacteria in the Intestine Drives TH1 Cell Induction and Inflammation," *Science* 358, no. 6361 (2017): 359–365, https://doi.org/10.1126/science.aan4526.

GLUTEN AND GUT

Whenever I speak about the mouth-and-bowel-disease connection, I inevitably get questions about gluten: "Does gluten do this? How does gluten do that? Should I eat this or that with gluten in it?" Here's the deal with gluten: the gluten protein (found in wheat) is provocative to certain people's immune systems, similar to how some people are lactose intolerant. For these people, the gluten protein is unable to be broken down and digested. So when this flood of "invading proteins" comes through the digestive system, the immune system activates an inflammatory response, with its army of white blood cells, to go and attack the nondigested gluten, as it's supposed to. And guess who's leading the charge? None other than MMP-8. Being that this happens in the gut, MMP-8 ends up cutting through the digestive tract, allowing the gluten and everything else to escape into the body. Basically, it is another version of leaky gut syndrome, which is really just inflammatory bowel disease. When I see patients with inflamed gums, I suggest refraining from gluten. It can't hurt, and there are no health benefits to gluten.

LEAKY GUT

Despite this book being about the mouth-body connection, I guess I've mentioned leaky gut syndrome enough times now to warrant an actual explanation.

Within the medical community, leaky gut is referred to as "increased intestinal permeability" and is often used in the context of digestive and stomach issues. To get an idea of what's going on inside with leaky gut syndrome, think of your intestines as the internal plumbing of your home, specifically the toilet. Toilets carry waste (whatever your body doesn't use) out of the house and to the sewer. Just like with your home's sewer system, you don't want the waste on the inside of those pipes touching *anything* on the outside (which is why plumbers are paid so well).

The reason is that this waste is toxic—it contains bacteria, toxins, fungi, you name it. If you had even a pinprick in your colon, all that crap (literally) would get into your body, and you'd die of sepsis. This is the reason why people who have colon surgery need a colostomy bag afterward: the bag allows the poop to bypass the colon while it heals. Leaky gut basically causes the same problem. When leaky gut occurs, the cells of the intestinal lining no longer tightly fit together, leaving gaps and becoming permeable.

Leaky gut syndrome happens in a number of ways:

- A damaged intestinal lining becomes too permeable. Larger, undigested food particles (like gluten proteins) and intestinal microbes escape into the bloodstream.
- Any food particles that leak into the bloodstream are viewed by the immune system as foreign bodies, and the immune system reacts with an inflammatory response.
- Microbes escape into the bloodstream, causing more immune system reactions. These microbes are often gram-negative gut bacteria whose outer membranes contain molecules called lipopolysaccharides (LPS). Lipopolysaccharides trigger the immune system even more.
- An activated immune system produces antibodies that can travel in the bloodstream and create an inflammatory response in other parts of the body, including joints, leading to arthritic pain and swelling.

When the toxic waste in our intestines leaks out into our abdominal cavities, all kinds of ailments come about. To name a few, we have low energy, bloating, discomfort, gas, diarrhea, and constipation ("Hey! Pepto Bismol!").

But the main point is that what happens in the gut also happens in the mouth; the tissues are the same, so the same "leakiness" occurs. This is why so many people with periodontal disease (now being called "leaky gums") also have gut issues. From chronic inflammation, that same MMP-8 enzyme that blows holes through our gums cuts through our intestines as well; the two systems are interconnected, and the mouth is at the top. So please take care of your mouth. Take some oral probiotics and see your dentist regularly.

ARTHRITIS

You may have noticed that one of the symptoms of leaky gut was "arthritic pain and swelling." Yep, arthritis is an inflammatory disease, and you better believe it can be caused indirectly by bacteria.

There are two main types of arthritis (creeky, painful joints). The first is osteoarthritis, which is usually associated with aging and usually affects one joint at a time (I have a bad knee). The other, rheumatoid arthritis (RA), is an autoimmune disease where the body attacks most or all of its joint spaces. Why this happens remains unknown, but discoveries are beginning to uncover what causes this systemic attack, and it seems to start with the mouth. New studies are showing that arthritis will occur when some of the microbes that escape the intestines cause systemic inflammation. These are the bacteria Pg, Fn, Pc, and Ec (among others).[37]

---

[37] Carol Torgan, "Gut Microbes Linked to Rheumatoid Arthritis," *NIH Research Matters*, National Institutes of Health, November 25, 2013, https://www.nih.gov/news-events/nih-research-matters/gut-microbes-linked-rheumatoid-arthritis.

These bacteria create antibodies that trigger inflammation and attack everything, including the lining of our joints, leading to inflammation and arthritis. Infected joints will then have the immune system constantly attack the joint spaces, creating inflammation in the form of osteoarthritis, rheumatoid arthritis, and gout. And to bring everything full circle, researchers are examining the poop of untreated RA patients and finding that 75 percent of them have bacteria present in their poop, compared to their healthy counterparts.[38]

The connection between mouth/gut health and arthritis is well known; when we are unable to process our food properly (see leaky gut above), we develop chronic systemic inflammation, which causes these arthritic complications. To combat this, we need to reduce the amount of these bad bacteria and increase our good bacteria to quiet our immune systems. This is primarily done by eating a healthy, plant-based whole-food diet and by having good oral health so that bacteria can't set up their residence in the mouth (the body) in the first place. Oh, let's not forget fiber. Fiber helps to clean our gut and move out toxins. Only 7 percent of people get enough fiber daily, which is recommended at 30 grams per day on average.[39]

THE MOUTH-INFLAMMATORY DISEASE CONNECTION

Periodontal disease (PD) is a massively widespread oral condition that majorly affects our overall health, now seen even in our poop and in arthritis. Because PD is asymptomatic in its early stages, it's often overlooked when unexplained ailments

---

38   Torgan, "Gut Microbes Linked to Rheumatoid Arthritis."

39   ASN Staff, "Most Americans Are Not Getting Enough Fiber in Our Diets," American Society for Nutrition, June 9, 2021, https://nutrition.org/most-americans-are-not-getting-enough-fiber-in-our-diets.

arise, allowing for our natural inflammatory response to spread to the rest of the body.

While some have healthy, strong, and controlled immune systems and will be able to fight off oral bacteria with relative ease, others will not. Those with underlying health issues and/or poor habits (e.g., stress, smoking, mediocre diets) or who are cursed with mutated inflammatory genes are already experiencing an inflamed state, and their bodies will undergo a heightened response—meaning that the same bacteria types and levels could be seen in multiple people, while their clinical presentations could be completely different.

Gingivitis, the curable precursor to periodontitis, is inflammation of the gingival tissues that has not yet destroyed the bone surrounding the teeth.

The key to combating this is knowledge, the knowledge that I'm giving you. By being aware of the implications of unchecked oral bacteria, you now know you do not have to not suffer like many of my unfortunate patients. But you do have to go see your dentist.

So far I've spoken about oral health and inflammation as it relates to one individual's systemic health. But as we'll see in the next chapter, it can be a family thing.

We're going to talk about something that's *super* important to me: babies! I want to share with you how oral bacteria can affect making, growing, and having children.

CHAPTER 7

Making Babies

THIS IS PROBABLY ONE OF MY FAVORITE STORIES. I HAD a young Hispanic couple (in their twenties) come into my practice on the advice of their obstetrician—they had been trying to conceive, without success, and their doctor had noticed that she (the wife) had a severe gum infection. At the time, I was one of the few dentists in Colorado performing salivary diagnostic testing on their patients (this was pure coincidence, as their obstetrician didn't know me from Eve and had merely advised them to "go see their dentist"). The couple was lucky that this was the case.

After we went through the normal checkup routine and I had confirmed the mouth infection, we spoke for a while. They told me the story of how they were wanting a baby. I explained how bacteria in the mouth can affect fertility (soon I'll be able to just point patients to this book). I also brought up the new salivary exams and how they could detect if those certain fertility-inhibiting bacteria were present. Without me even having to ask, they wanted the test.

I first conducted the saliva exam and then performed the

perio and gum disease treatment, which she desperately needed. I gave the test to the husband also—if he had the same bacteria, she could be reinfected easily by their kissing or eating with the same fork after one another. It turned out that they both had sky-high levels of Fn (the main culprit with infertility). Both left my office only after receiving vital periodontal therapy (a good, deep Fn treatment) along with a prescription for antibiotics.

Three months later they were pregnant.

Was this a coincidence? Maybe. But you might think differently after all I share with you on the mouth-fertility connection. Regardless, the story still gives me warm fuzzies.

Let's look at all the ways the mouth can affect reproduction.

THE MOUTH AND FEMALE FERTILITY ISSUES (AND SOME MALE ONES TOO)

Confession time: I'm a fairly passionate person when it comes to oral health (if you couldn't tell already), but I turn it up a notch when it comes to oral health and reproductive issues. Reproduction is a fundamental right to all, and the fact that something as simple as oral health can hamper that really gets under my skin. So there's my impetus for you. But let's look at more of the science behind the connection, especially for us ladies (I'll include some for the guys also, as it takes two to tango).

LADIES FIRST

The mouth affects reproduction in two major ways: infertility or difficult conception and pregnancy outcomes. This is largely attributed to the Fn and Pg oral bacteria. Fn is widely known to cross the placenta in pregnancy, causing developmental issues, and Pg creates problems in trying to conceive. In fact, gum disease in women has been shown to have the same magnitude of negative effects on trying to conceive as obesity, both increasing the time frame of getting pregnant by two months (seven months versus five months in the healthy population).[40] But beyond that and my anecdotal story, try these facts on for size:

- Fn infection causes a three times greater risk of infertility.
- Fn, via MMP-8, causes an increased risk for preterm and low birth weight. (Its metabolic waste products cause fetal toxicity after crossing the placenta—more on that later.)[41]
- Chronic inflammation from perio affects fertility by preventing ovulation and implantation of the embryo or not sustaining its implantation.
- Perio disease can affect the success probability of infertility treatments as it leads to bacteremia, endotoxemia, cytokines, and increased immunity to heat shock proteins, all of which have been associated with reproductive failure.[42]
- Salivary Pg is connected to difficult conception in young women. The hormones used in assisted reproductive therapies were found to increase gingival inflammation and periodontal degradation (tissue loss), both of which place patients in a chronically inflamed state that decreases the chances of conception.[43]
- Chronic periodontitis is linked with known causes of

40   Hanna Hanssen, "Gum Disease Can Increase the Time It Takes to Become Pregnant," PR Web, press release, July 5, 2011, https://www.prweb.com/releases/2011/7/prweb8618711.htm.

41   M. Cenk Haytaç, Turan Cetin, and Gulash Seydaoglu, "The Effects of Ovulation Induction during Infertility Treatment on Gingival Inflammation," *Journal of Periodontology* 75, no. 6 (June 2004): 805–810, https://doi.org/10.1902/jop.2004.75.6.805.

42   Haytaç, Cetin, and Seydaoglu, "The Effects of Ovulation Induction."

43   Susanna Paju et al., "*Porphyromonas gingivalis* May Interfere with Conception in Women," *Journal of Oral Microbiology* 9, no. 1 (2017), https://doi.org/10.1080/20002297.2017.1330644.

infertility, such as endometriosis and pelvic inflammatory disease.[44]

Are you convinced yet? Let me lay another on you. Chronic inflammation impedes women's ability to ovulate; just the mere presence of inflammation (often originating in the mouth, as we've learned) affects the release of the egg and the implantation of an embryo. And we haven't gotten to what happens *if* you can get pregnant. But let's take a break and talk to the guys for a moment.

FOR THE FELLAS

Around 10 percent of the population suffers from infertility, which is most often thought to be on the part of the woman. However, the truth is it's about half and half! As far as male infertility and the mouth goes, it's about what you'd expect; bacteria in the mouth move to the body and cause a heap of problems.

In particular, perio disease affects the ability to achieve an erection—the consequences on reproduction are obvious. This happens because of Pg, as Pg decreases the production of arginine, which is the precursor to nitric oxide: the vasodilator (artery widener) that is responsible for "raising the flag."

Beyond hampering the mechanics of sexual reproduction in men, poor oral hygiene also drastically affects sperm, a key ingredient to baby-making, in terms of count and mobility. (Conversely, the right perio treatments will undo whatever

---

44   Shahryar K. Kavoussi et al., "Periodontal Disease and Endometriosis: Analysis of the National Health and Nutrition Examination Survey," *Fertility and Sterility* 91, no. 2 (February 2009): 335–342, https://doi.org/10.1016/j.fertnstert.2007.12.075; Allison McKinnon et al., "A Case of Adolescent Pelvic Inflammatory Disease Caused by a Rare Bacterium: *Fusobacterium nucleatum,*" *Journal of Pediatric & Adolescent Gynecology* 26, no. 6 (December 2013): e113–e115, https://doi.org/10.1016/j.jpag.2013.02.008.

damage was done.)[45] This happens via bacteriospermia (bacteria in the sperm), which can originate from an oral cavity infection. These bacteria kill sperm, reducing the overall count and reducing the mobility of the surviving sperm by changing their shape (morphology). Lastly, men with gum infections have been found to have the IL-6 gene mutation in their seminal fluid, which, amongst all its other terrible effects, is also associated with infertility (as mentioned before, IL-6 makes its host chronically inflamed).

Surely you can see the picture forming now. You can get pregnant *if* the egg is released and *if* the sperm count is high enough and *if* they can even swim that far and *if* the egg becomes fertilized and *if* the fertilized egg attaches to the uterus. The odds of that happening are already slim enough. Throw in an oral infection or gene mutation, and you're looking at the possibly impossible.

ONE STEP FORWARD, TWO STEPS BACK

You might be thinking, "Well, I can see how oral health affects the tried-and-true method of sexual reproduction, but what about using today's technology to assist with pregnancy? Don't they have drugs that help me ovulate?" Good idea, but there are problems here as well. Plus, remember, our goal is *total* health, and the body's systems all affect one another—we don't want everything else to be fine while we ignore the one part of us that is ill. Change your mind to start looking at the body more holistically.

Two of the more popular methods of assisted reproduc-

---

45   Emily Brockette, "Infertility and Inflammation: The Potential Connection to Periodontal Disease," Dentistry IQ, May 21, 2018, www.dentistryiq.com/dental-hygiene/student-hygiene/article/16367898/infertility-and-inflammation-the-potential-connection-to-periodontal-disease.

tive therapy (ART) are in vitro fertilization (IVF), where the egg is fertilized in a lab and then placed into the woman, and intrauterine insemination (IUI—*those fertility specialists sure love their acronyms*), where the sperm is directly implanted— via medical procedure—into the woman while she's ovulating. These methods are solid, but they require the use of medications that assist with fertility and ovulation, in particular prescription hormones, such as estrogen and progesterone.

But here's the rub. Those medications cause increased gingival inflammation, and without addressing the root issue, *you'll only release more oral bacteria into the bloodstream.* You know the drill by now: more bacteria only leads to a chronically inflamed state that horribly reduces the chances of conception.

If you are undergoing ART without having addressed your oral health, I advise you to stop and receive the necessary gum disease screening and, if needed, gum infection treatment from your dentist first. It's also important to note that when you do this, you will have increased levels of bacteria in your blood for a short time from having everything in your mouth stirred up (a necessary evil for healing). Because of this, I also advise that you wait at least one month after a perio treatment before reattempting ART, just to let everything calm down. Trust me, I know the idea of pausing to wait is not something most people going through fertility treatments want to hear. I know that because, having gone through it, I am familiar with the process myself.

PREGNANCY, DELIVERY, AND ORAL HEALTH

While there should be cause to celebrate if you become pregnant despite the difficulties associated with poor oral hygiene, your problems won't stop simply because you've conceived. In fact, you could say they've only just begun.

Poor oral hygiene before pregnancy almost unerringly becomes worse after pregnancy, typically for a few simple reasons. For starters, the pregnancy hormones, estrogen and progesterone, dilate your blood vessels, increasing blood flow (this is how your baby gets the nutrients they need and also why you're so swollen). The problem here is that this increase in blood volume increases gingival inflammation and bleeding gums (just as with ART drugs), making it easier for bacteria to spread all over the body. And not just your body this time but your baby's also. I see this all the time with pregnant women in my office—their gums are a hot mess and, by default, super-*duper* leaky.

Next, it's common for women to experience nausea, vomiting, and all the typical morning sickness symptoms while pregnant. This gives a reason for a patient to not desire to brush their teeth (per the gag reflex). This, plus frequent upchucking dissolving your teeth in stomach acid, makes for a perfect storm of cavities and gum disease. Lastly, every person that's ever cared for a pregnant woman is familiar with the midnight ice cream cravings—sweets and carbs don't help the situation either. You can see how all of this tees up everything oral bacteria need to make a grand slam on your body.

But like I said, it's not just your body this time. Oral bacteria, once they get out of the mouth, can do significant harm to your baby. MMP-8 due to bacterial infection causes preterm delivery by rupturing membranes, and Fn causes stillbirths.[46] What occurs is that bacteria make their way down to the placenta and work themselves inside the gestational membranes. Our immune systems, responding to the infection, flood the area with white blood cells and MMP-8. MMP-8 cuts through tissue

---

46   Mayo Clinic, "Premature Birth: Symptoms and Causes," accessed April 25, 2023, https://www.mayoclinic. org/diseases-conditions/premature-birth/symptoms-causes/syc-20376730.

indiscriminately, thus perforating the amniotic sac, "breaking your water," and creating an early delivery. If the bacteria happen to be Fn (or Pg also), the toxic metabolic waste products from that bacteria can cause stillbirth. But don't just take my word for it. Consider the following:

- Women with periodontal disease have a 30–50% higher chance of having a preterm delivery or an infant with a low birth weight.[47]
- If you treat perio by the second trimester, you reduce your risk of preterm birth from 14.7 percent to 9.7 percent.[48]
- 40 percent of pregnant women have some form of perio disease.[49]
- As compared to mothers with healthy gums who deliver premature and underweight babies, pregnant women with gingivitis are three times more likely, those with chronic gum disease are four to seven times more likely, and those with moderate chronic perio are eight times more likely to do the same.[50]

---

47   Rajiv Saini, Santosh Saini, and Sugandha R. Saini, "Periodontitis: A Risk for Delivery of Premature Labor and Low-Birth-Weight Infants," Journal of Natural Science, Biology and Medicine 1, no. 1 (July 2012): 40-2, doi:10.4103/0976-9668.71672.

48   Nikolaos P. Polyzos, et al., "Effect of Periodontal Disease Treatment during Pregnancy on Preterm Birth Incidence: A Metaanalysis of Randomized Trials," AJOG 200, no. 3 (March 2009): 225–232, https://doi.org/10.1016/j.ajog.2008.09.020.

49   Piaopiao Chen, Feiruo Hong, and Xuefen Yu, "Prevalence of Periodontal Disease in Pregnancy: A Systematic Review and Meta-Analysis," Journal of Dentistry 125, (October 2022): 104253, https://doi.org/10.1016/j.jdent.2022.104253.

50   Marjorie K. Jeffcoat et al., "Periodontal Infection and Preterm Birth: Results of a Prospective Study," Journal of the American Dental Association 132, no. 7 (July 2001): 875–880, https://doi.org/10.14219/jada.archive.2001.0299; "Dental Care and Pregnancy" WebMD, March 4, 2022, https://www.webmd.com/oral-health/dental-care-pregnancy#:~:text=Don't%20let%20the%20word,who%20also%20have%20pregnancy%20gingivitis.

- PD leads to preeclampsia, premature rupture of membranes, C-section, and preterm delivery.[51]

Premature births are before thirty-seven weeks and are associated with the following conditions:

- Respiratory issues (asthma, reduced lung capacity)
- Heart issues (patent ductus arteriosus, hypotension, heart murmurs, heart failure)
- Brain issues (intraventricular hemorrhage)
- Difficulty regulating body temperature due to low stored fat
- GI issues
- Blood issues (anemia and jaundice)
- Metabolism issues (hypoglycemia, premature glucose metabolizing system)
- Immature immune system (infection prone)
- Cerebral palsy
- Cognitive/learning delays and behavioral problems
- Vision and hearing problems
- Dental issues (delayed eruption, missing teeth, misaligned teeth, discolored teeth)
- SIDS

Needless to say, I bet there are some others out there, like me, that are gobsmacked by the lack of professional awareness in this area. So for the sake of yourself and your little one, take care of your mouth (and your baby daddy's).

---

51   Rajiv Saini, Santosh Saini, and Sugandha R. Saini, "Periodontitis: A Risk for Delivery of Premature Labor and Low Birth Weight Infants," Journal of Natural Science, *Biology and Medicine* 2, no. 1 (January 2011): 50–52, https://doi.org/10.4103/0976-9668.71672.

I'd like to address the "old wives' tale" that it's bad for you to go see the dentist when you're pregnant. I don't how that got started, but it's the furthest thing from the truth, and after reading those statistics, I hope you can see that your dentist is actually the one you *want* to be visiting during pregnancy.

I do understand that pregnant women grow tired of being poked, prodded, examined, X-rayed, and so on. And yes, no dental treatment (or any treatment, really) is going to be 100 percent safe during pregnancy, but still, it's certainly better to get it done sooner rather than later, especially with the risks involved. And hey, *it's for your baby, right?* Once, I had a pregnant woman who reluctantly came into my office, gave me an attitude, and put up resistance when I suggested an X-ray, only to have me finally convince her and reveal the nasty hidden abscess that had been leaking harmful bacteria to her baby for God knows how long—*and I'm the bad guy?* But even if you're unconvinced, you can at least come and get the treatment you need *before* you start growing a life, yeah?

One last falsehood I'd like to correct is that some of my pregnant patients think they don't need to come to see me if they "just have gingivitis" and not "gum disease." If you're unaware, the difference between the two is that while gingivitis is just swollen gums, gum disease is actual bone loss. As far as the mouth is concerned, there is an obvious difference in severity. But for the point at hand, there is *zero* difference—*they both cause leaky gums and let bacteria hurt you and your baby.* Plus gingivitis, when left unchecked, turns into gum disease, and you can't cure bone loss because bone *loss* means there's *nothing there to cure.* Meanwhile, the treatments for gingivitis are plentiful. Are you scheduling your next appointment yet?

GESTATIONAL DIABETES

You saw this one coming. I've already connected diabetes to the mouth, and now I've connected the mouth to pregnancy complications. So you'd better bet I'm going to link it to gestational diabetes too.

Gestational diabetes mellitus (GDM) is diabetes that occurs during pregnancy. In only 10 percent of cases are the moms prediabetic, meaning they were already showing signs of insulin resistance before they got pregnant. And believe it or not, it is the most common complication of pregnancy. This occurs when the placental hormones (estrogen, cortisol, and placental lactogen) are secreted and block the effects of insulin, leading to insulin resistance (diabetes). The further along you are in pregnancy, the larger the placenta grows and the more of these hormones you produce, which is why most GDM is diagnosed during the third trimester. This, in the end, causes 30 to 50 percent of women to develop type 2 diabetes within five years postpartum. While there hasn't been an exact study on the relationship here, consider this, and the fact that periodontal disease already exacerbates diabetic issues, and you've got yourself the ultimate double whammy.

RETURN ON INVESTMENT

So beyond improving fertility, avoiding diabetes, and...you know...*saving your baby's life*, you can save yourself a chunk of change too with oral care! The major cost associated with all I've been describing here is time spent in the hospital, especially for premature babies that need to stay in the NICU for months on end. Take another look at the list of conditions preterm babies suffer from and convert it into dollar signs—if you won't go see your dentist, at least check up on your medical plan.

Mothers with atypical births will need to go to the hospital sooner also, increasing the total time under care and the associated cost. Don't forget that, due to PD, Mom can also develop a form of pregnancy hypertension called preeclampsia (*coins jingling*), have a C-section (*piggy banks breaking*), and God forbid, any would-be-avoided type-2 diabetes (*cha-ching!*).

To quantify this a bit, check out these numbers:[52]

- Compared to atypical pregnancies, "normal" births had 40 percent lower overall costs and 9 percent fewer hospitalizations.
- Pregnant women who completed perio treatment saved $2,433 in annual medical costs.
- Pregnant perio patients (*Sally sells seashells…*), if treated during pregnancy, saw a 74 percent reduction in medical costs: $866 versus $3,299 (atypical pregnancy–related medical costs).
- Type 2 diabetes patients saw a 40 percent reduction in costs and a 39 percent reduction in hospitalizations when treated for perio.

I don't think you need much more than all that. For the sake of you, your baby, and your pocketbook, go see your dentist.

THE MOUTH-FERTILITY CONNECTION

Suffice it to say, that young couple did right coming to see me when they did. The science behind her and his oral bacterial infections hurting their chances of conceiving is solid. So I feel

---

52 Marjorie K. Jeffcoat et al., "Impact of Periodontal Therapy on General Health: Evidence from Insurance Data for Five Systemic Conditions," *American Journal of Preventive Medicine* 47, no. 2 (August 2014): 166–174, https://doi.org/10.1016/j.amepre.2014.04.001.

comfortable in saying that the odds of her becoming pregnant after my treatment being a coincidence are slim. I don't say that to toot my own horn but to herald this amazing truth of how oral health can improve people's overall lives in ways they would have never thought. And I say it to applaud the couple for being willing to listen to "unconventional wisdom" in order to be fully healthy. While proper oral hygiene won't solve your every problem, I wish that people would come to this mouth-body connection realization sooner because there's so much it *can* fix. But sometimes it takes trying everything and everything failing before coming to the truth. It is what it is, and this journey is worth it.

Whew! Almost got emotional there. I think I'd better take a breather, which, funny enough, is what the next chapter is about: breath!

CHAPTER 8

Careful! Don't Swallow Your Own Tongue

I KNOW I'VE BEEN HITTING YOU HARD ON THE WHOLE "OMG, there's bacteria in my mouth, and I need a dentist right now" rhetoric, so let's take a look at the mouth-body connection from another angle. The mouth can still affect your overall health without the adverse assistance of bacteria. One of the most prominent ways is with your breathing (Makes sense, right? You have to breathe to live, and *air comes through the mouth*.) Let me tell you the story of Maria and how I, as a dentist, was able to help her breathe at night and avoid an early grave.

Maria, another long-term patient of mine, came to me one day for her routine checkup. She was one of those cute little older ladies that took care of themselves and was *always* dressed to the nines (appearance was high on her list of priorities). But similar to how most of my stories start, that day Maria was looking *rough*, to say the least. She was pale, had bags under her eyes, and was extremely lethargic—basically, she looked as though she'd been hit by a bus and nothing like how I was accustomed to seeing her (usually I'm a little jealous, but today was the exception). When I got her in the chair, I immediately noticed her bad breath (also uncommon for her). I set down my dental mirror and asked her what was going on. She shared that she hadn't been sleeping well and was waking up with acid reflux and chest pain, which she described as the sensation of something sitting on her chest. (This is what people on the verge of a heart attack usually say.) "I feel like I'm going to die," was her cry for help.

I asked why she hadn't seen her primary care physician, and she told me she had called him, saying it was an emergency, but that he wasn't available for another *six* weeks. I let her know that, while I wasn't a physician, she was exhibiting symptoms of obstructive sleep apnea (OSA), and my office could test her for it right away. Scared for her life, she obviously agreed, and within a few days, she had completed her sleep test. I partnered with a board-certified sleep physician to review her results, and as I had suspected, her results were off the chart.

She tested positive for severe sleep apnea with an oxygen desaturation level of 72 percent—anything below 90 percent is concerning, and below 80 percent means you're losing brain cells or ready for a heart attack (Maria wasn't exaggerating about feeling close to death). She stopped breathing more than thirty times per hour! We partnered with her physician, and the good news was that her issue could be treated with a mandibular advancement device (a mouth guard–looking thing, more on that later) in combination with a CPAP machine. We took her measurements and got her in the appliance ASAP. Within two weeks, Maria was right as rain.

And there you have it. A simple tool that adjusted my patient's mouth improved her overall health and quality of life tenfold. She had no more pain in her chest or headaches, and her sleep was *way* better (she did get her heart checked out and everything was normal). In this chapter, the problem I'll focus on isn't so much a matter of a particular bacterium, as in the other chapters, as it is the mouth's structure and the mechanics of how we breathe when we sleep, both of which can drastically affect our overall health.

ALL KINDS OF APNEA

Apnea is a condition that causes you to stop breathing while sleeping and comes in two main varieties: central and obstructive. Central sleep apnea (CSA) is basically when the brain forgets to tell your body to breathe while you sleep. (Come on brain—get it together!) Treatments for CSA include medications, weaning off opioid medications, continuous positive airway pressure (CPAP)—like devices, and phrenic nerve stimulation.

Obstructive sleep apnea (OSA)—the type we'll be focusing on—is much less complicated, though maybe a bit more disturbing. OSA occurs when our airway collapses and becomes "obstructed." Typically, during sleep, a patient's tongue will fall back and choke the patient, thus collapsing the airway and causing the patient to apply effort in breathing to bypass the obstruction (force the airway back open)—with this, you may already be seeing why CPAP devices are used. Because a sufferer of OSA is essentially being choked to death, the heart rate jumps up in response to the lessening oxygen levels (usually below 80 percent during an obstructive bout), signaling that something needs to be done. In an effort to save itself from being asphyxiated, our body will send a rush of adrenaline to the brain stem to wake us up and start breathing once more (again with the whole "need air to live" thing). What this means is that those with OSA are waking up multiple times *per hour* to keep from kicking the bucket during their beauty rest.

Because OSA is based on airway collapsibility, it doesn't only occur with obese people, as typically assumed. Formerly, it was thought that OSA was only seen in either athletes with short, thick necks or those who were morbidly obese and had similar builds. But now we are seeing OSA more in older, thin, postmenopausal women. You can also imagine how airway collapsibility occurs in these patients. After menopause, women lose bone mass. Less bone mass means there are fewer places for skin, muscles, and tendons to hold on to, making the airway more prone to collapsing. Plus, as we grow older, the tonicity of our muscles, skin, and cartilage declines, meaning our airway doesn't have enough strength to stay open anyhow. (Translation: just because you were in the clear with OSA two years ago doesn't mean you are fine today.) Another commonly held falsehood is that OSA only affects those who snore. Here are a few other facts for you:[53]

- 85 percent of patients with diabetes have OSA.
- 80 percent of people with sleep apnea are undiagnosed; it's believed one in five Americans have OSA.
- OSA patients who receive treatment will save approximately $200,000 in medical bills over a lifetime by avoiding comorbidities.
- Untreated sleep apnea is worse for your health than smoking cigarettes.
- Untreated mild or moderate sleep apnea will take fifteen years off your life on average.

53   Medoville Inc. Medical Supplies, "The Dangers of Obstructive Sleep Apnea," blog post, January 28, 2019, https://medoville.com/the-dangers-of-obstructive-sleep-apnea/.

- Severe sleep apnea is fatal (a matter of time).
- People with severe sleep apnea have a three times greater risk of dying from a stroke than those without.
- Mild to moderate OSA patients have a 50 percent greater mortality risk from sudden death between 10:00 p.m. and 6:00 a.m. than those without OSA.
- 20 percent of all vehicle accidents are caused by excessive daytime sleepiness, which can be attributed to OSA.
- Drivers who slept only four or five hours have crash rates "similar to the U.S. government's estimates of the risk associated with driving with a blood alcohol concentration equal to or slightly above the legal limit for alcohol in the U.S."[54]
- Even with only getting six hours of sleep, compared to the recommended seven or eight, you are inhibited to the same degree as being legally drunk.

Sleep apnea can affect your life in ways you've never considered. Obviously, not breathing can have some drastic consequences, but there are also some serious side effects to a chronic lack of sleep. Let's take a look at how important sleep is.

THE IMPORTANCE OF SLEEP

I can hear it already: "What's the big deal with sleep? I've got kids, and they wake me up all the time, and I'm okay." Or my favorite: "I just don't sleep that much." Yeah, you don't, and yeah, *you should*. For starters, similarly to how our immune system uses the lymphatic system to wash our bodies of trash (toxins) to protect our immunity, our brains use the glymphatic

---

54 Jaclyn Trop, "Drowsy Driving: Worse than Drunk Driving?" *US News and World Report*, December 15, 2016, https://cars.usnews.com/cars-trucks/advice/best-cars-blog/2016/12/drowsy-driving-worse-than-drunk-driving.

system to wash toxins from there. That cleanup happens at night while we sleep—all the toxins that make their way to our brains during the day are flushed out every night by this system, and if you're not sleeping, those toxins start accumulating. Obviously, this process has implications for dementia and Alzheimer's. Also, in developing children (yep, kids can have sleep apnea too), the growth hormone is released only during sleep. It's *super* important for little ones to get the sleep they need to grow appropriately.

I want to look a little more closely at the structure of our sleep so that we can understand more clearly how and why sleep apnea jacks it all up.

SLEEP CYCLES AND OSA

Our sleep cycle is characterized by two types of sleep: non-rapid eye movement (NREM) and rapid eye movement (REM). The basic structure of our slumber is NREM 1, 2, 3, and then 4, followed by REM (this is known as sleep architecture). This pattern repeats throughout the night, with the REM cycle growing longer on each iteration.

NREM is our "deep sleep." This is when there is minimal brain activity and we heal and recover from illnesses—it's what helps us feel "rested." Early in the night, NREM is the main chunk of our rest, but as we continue sleeping, REM becomes the larger portion, starting in the early morning. Though it may not seem like it, REM sleep is the most important stage of sleep—this is when the brain is *very active* and where dreams occur (ironically, this is also where most sleep apnea occurs). Think about the times at night when you are partly awake, partly asleep, and dreaming—that's your REM sleep.

When in REM sleep, we become paralyzed, which is to our

benefit, lest we'd be acting out our mental images of running, fighting, and attempting to fly. Considering our nightly bouts of paralysis, you can easily see why OSA most often occurs in REM sleep—everything relaxes, and our airway collapses; meanwhile, we can't move. This falls right in line with those that pass away in their sleep; autopsies performed on these people consistently show that the time of death falls between two and six o'clock in the morning, right in the REM sleep realm. The mechanics behind this are as follows: an obstruction occurs, paralysis prevents correction of the obstruction, too much pressure is placed on the heart or brain, a heart attack or stroke happens, and the patient never wakes up.

People who sleepwalk have a disconnection where they don't experience paralysis while in REM sleep.

MORE ISSUES WITH INTERRUPTED SLEEP

Being that OSA occurs mostly during REM sleep, it also interrupts our dreams. Why does this matter, you ask? It's because dreams are what help us solidify anything we've learned that day, lock memories in place, and erase anxiety and fear. A common connection with those who habitually wake up in REM sleep is anxiety—if you can't sleep and erase your fears, you'll naturally be more afraid when you're awake. And anxiety isn't something to be taken mildly; it can and does lead to other medical conditions.

Sleep problems and anxiety are both increasingly seen in post-menopausal women, who, "coincidentally," are at a higher risk of sleep apnea.

Sleep also affects our diet. While we sleep, the hormones responsible for hunger, leptin and ghrelin, are released. If we aren't sleeping, these hormones become disrupted, and the following day we're starving. I'm not just speaking for myself here. When we don't get a good night's rest, we tend to have poor appetite control the next day and are drawn to carbs and sugary snacks for quick energy fixes (poor sleep is directly related to poor glucose and weight control). Meanwhile, obesity and type 2 diabetes are both contributing factors for OSA, as 83 percent of diabetics have sleep apnea, whether they know it or not. This may be a matter of the chicken or the egg: which came first, OSA or type 2?[55]

Another hormone involved with apnea is cortisol, the stress hormone. When we stop breathing, our bodies sense that we are choking and dying, so they send a cortisol spike to wake us up out of our paralysis and kick everything back on. In addition to creating inflammation, as mentioned in Chapter 1, when cortisol is chronically high, it lowers our immune response, which is exactly why, when people don't sleep well for a few days, they wind up getting sick. This continual supply of stress hormones puts our bodies into a fight-or-flight response when our sympathetic system pushes out those stress hormones. If chronic, a patient will never return to the parasympathetic rest-and-digest stage, setting them up for illness. This is also connected to daytime indigestion and constipation, to premature aging (oxidative stress), and—back again—to weight control and anxiety issues.

All this would make you think that people who are constantly waking up would take notice. Well, it's not so simple. Typically, you need to be awake for three or more minutes to

---

55   Sushmita Pamidi and Esra Tasali, "Obstructive Sleep Apnea and Type 2 Diabetes: Is There a Link?," *Frontiers in Neurology* 3 (August 2012): 126, https://doi.org/10.3389/fneur.2012.00126.

remember that you've woken up. The nature of having OSA is that people will jostle awake for only a few seconds, meaning it's entirely possible to wake up fifty, sixty, or *seventy* times an hour, be completely exhausted, and think that you slept the night through. So, while you may be "sleeping like a trucker," you may not be getting through all the sleep stages, especially the REM stage, where the real rest is done.

OSA TELLS

My treatment coordinator, Kim, was in her thirties and was suffering. She was always tired and had consistent TMJ head-aches (we'll discuss these later) and brain fog. She had bruxism (teeth grinding) to the point where her teeth were breaking; we even tried root canals and crowns, but she broke those as well. She was forgetting her routine tasks and constantly calling in sick. Needless to say, her performance was declining at work.

I easily recognized the symptoms and suggested she take a sleep test, and sure enough, she had a severe case of sleep apnea. We pinpointed the issue to be originating from her adenoids, and she had them removed last April. This procedure is horribly painful for an adult, but Kim was desperate. Since then, she's recovered and is now sleeping well with no more headaches. Her overall health and job performance have drastically improved.

I was able to recognize the signs of sleep apnea and got Kim the help she needed. I'd like to go over some of the other signs of sleep apnea in order to arm you with the same knowledge and allow you to help others as well as yourself.

ANATOMY AND GENETICS

Anytime a person has a short or shortened jaw, it sets them

up for sleep apnea. An example is a "class II occlusion" where someone has a deep bite (think buckteeth). Another example is when people have their premolars removed for orthodontic purposes. Both of these examples "shorten the mouth" and make less room for the tongue (the tongue often is the culprit in blocking the airway, and less room increases the chances of obstruction). In the same fashion, a large or strong tongue can cause this issue. You can tell if someone has a large tongue by seeing whether or not it's "scalloped." A scalloped tongue occurs when a tongue is too big for a person's mouth and their teeth create indentations along its sides.

Fun fact! People who gag easily often have sleep apnea.

Naturally, because these factors are influenced by genetics, you can look at a family medical history to screen for sleep apnea. From obesity to diabetes to bone structure, epigenetics plays a large role in all diseases, and sleep apnea is no different.

TEETH GRINDING AND HEADACHES

Teeth grinding, known as bruxism, is as bad as it sounds: molars and incisors being clenched together and rubbed down until they break, exposing the nerve or, even worse, cracking the root (woof, gives me the willies). While this cringeworthy ailment has its connections to being overly stressed, it's also a sign of OSA. The reasoning is something similar to the point I made above with "short mouths." When someone's airway collapses, their brain (before it wakes them) sends a signal to jut the jaw forward and open up the passage (move the tongue forward)— essentially, your body puts your mouth in the same position as a mandibular appliance does (I'll talk more about these awesome tools under the treatment section). The problem is your teeth are pressed together when your brain sends this signal. To get a feel for how this hurts you, try this: bite down firmly and start rubbing your teeth together. Doesn't feel good, does it? Now imagine unconsciously doing that action potentially *hundreds of times a night*. Just the thought gives me more goosebumps. When someone comes into my office with flattened back teeth (like a cow's) and lots of wear on their front teeth, it's a dead giveaway for bruxism and, potentially, OSA.

But wait, there's more! If you are pressing and grinding your teeth all night, the muscles involved will be worn out and sore (think of it as working out all night). This is what's known as temporomandibular joint dysfunction (TMJ). You'll know where this joint is if you've ever had a super chewy meal or snack. The joint is right next to your ear, which is why when someone has a noisy joint, they will hear the popping loudly (minor sounds are not always an issue). There are two main muscles that help this joint function, the temporalis and masseter muscles. If you squeeze your teeth together, you can feel the temporalis protrude on the sides of your head, around the temple area. You'll really notice this if you're eating with someone who grinds their teeth—since they've been "working out all night," their temporal muscles will be *huge* and with every bite, their heads will bulge. The masseter muscles are located at the bottom corners of the jaw and will look like "jowls" in someone who overuses these muscles.

People with TMJ, especially men, will wake up with sore temples and/or headaches on the sides of their head. Meanwhile, people with sleep apnea will also wake up with headaches in the center of their forehead, which is directly due to oxygen deprivation.

Gastroesophageal reflux disease (GERD), or acid reflux, is *highly* correlated to sleep apnea (approximately 60 percent of all OSA patients have GERD).[56] Specifically, if a patient says their acid flex is worse when they lie down at night or when they wake up in the morning, they are more likely to have sleep apnea—acid reflux during the day (when we are upright) is more likely to be related to the foods we eat and indigestion.

Here's another experiment for you (having fun yet?): close your mouth shut, plug your nose, and try to breathe. Feel that vacuum sensation in your chest? That's your pyloric valve or sphincter muscle, which stops the contents of your stomach from going up your esophagus. This sphincter opens up when we eat and otherwise remains closed, except when upchucking, of course.

When we have an obstruction while sleeping, the positive pressure that occurs is strong enough to open the pyloric valve, and since you're lying down, all the contents of your stomach are free to move about the cabin, resulting in GERD. Making matters worse, chronic GERD erodes the base of the esophagus, which can cause the disorder called Barrett's esophagus. This condition, if you're unaware, often turns into cancer. Our stomach acid is only meant to be in our stomach, and with a continual wash of the corrosive fluid, the cells of our lower esophagus are changed and become precancerous. This can be fixed via surgery, but be sure not to wait around to fix your GERD issue. In addition, GERD erodes your teeth and turns them yellow, and you will have chronic bad breath no matter how many times you gargle mouthwash.

---

56   Sleep Center of Middle Tennessee, "GERD and Sleep Apnea: Treating OSA Helps Reduce Nighttime Reflux," *Sleep Center of Middle Tennessee* (blog), last updated October 25, 2022, https://sleepcenterinfo.com/blog/connection-gerd-sleep-apnea/.

Please don't misquote me; in no way am I about to say "OSA causes ADHD." However, you can't deny the connections that are there. It's well known that when you don't breathe while sleeping, your sympathetic system turns on and couples with cortisol release, which makes kids hyperactive and unable to concentrate when they are awake—the cortisol is too much for their bodies to handle. With this being the case, many times ADHD is misdiagnosed, and the problem actually lies in the child not breathing properly while sleeping. It's also not uncommon for children to grind their teeth at night. Coincidence?

This is largely due to the child's bone structure, whether it be their jaws not growing properly or just being too small. Amongst other reasons, improper growth can be attributed to poor tongue posture or oral habits, such as thumb-sucking. Proper tongue posture is such that when you're resting, your tongue is set on the anterior palate, just behind your two front teeth. In children, this pressure causes the palate to broaden and flatten, increasing the volume of their sinuses and allowing them to breathe better. Habits such as thumb-sucking cause breathing issues as the action places pressure on the palate, causing it to vault up into the sinuses and create the opposite effect.

However, because children are still young, the issues are easily fixable. Young people's bones are softer and more pliable—I always say, "We're like dinosaurs. The more time that goes by, the more our bones become like fossils." With some mild to moderate interference, you can easily redirect the growth pattern of children. This is also why it's so important to screen children for sleep apnea (more commonly thought to affect older and fatter people) when they exhibit sleeping problems, attention issues, teeth grinding, or any of the other issues mentioned here. Additionally, other signs include allergies, chronic sinus issues, and chronic ear infections.

Don't forget to look at your kids' adenoids. When they open their mouths, if you cannot see the back of their throat because their adenoids are "kissing/touching," they should see an ENT to discuss treatment.

AND MORE!

The rest of these don't really deserve a section of their own but are important nonetheless. For example, if someone is taking two or more blood pressure medications, the likelihood of them having sleep apnea is strong. Whether you're breathing or not, it's still your heart's job to circulate oxygenated blood, and when you have OSA, it puts immense pressure on your heart, as you can imagine. Many patients even experience their heart rate spiking uncontrollably during the night, and atrial fibrillation (A-fib) is usually associated with sleep apnea.

Know anyone who always seems to have a runny nose? Allergies and postnasal drip are often signs of sleep apnea. You see, nasal breathing, the healthy type of breathing, is essential because it quite literally filters the air we breathe; our nose hairs and cilia clean out all the dust and bacteria that we inhale as it passes through our nasal passages. However, a patient that has OSA is forced to breathe through their mouth to clear an obstruction, lest they choke to death. This bypasses our built-in filtration system and results in "year-round allergies."

Mouth tape is a great way to train your body to breathe through your nose. Ensure you do not have sleep apnea before trying this at night. I recommend using it during the day first, to get used to it before trying to sleep with it on.

This next one is fairly unique, I think. Oftentimes when I'm screening my patients for sleep apnea, I'll ask how frequently "they wake up to go pee in the night." Unerringly, I receive quizzical looks in response (probably just like the one you have right now). Here's why I ask: normally when we sleep, an antidiuretic hormone is released, which, obviously, lets us sleep through the night without running to the potty or soiling the sheets. Did you catch what I said? "Normally when we *sleep*." If you're constantly waking up from sleep apnea (whether you remember it or not), your body doesn't release said hormone; thus, you have to go tinkle more often.

If your child is chronically wetting the bed, this may be a sign of apnea.

And then there are all the obvious ones: bags under the eyes, slumped/tired posture, forward head posture, trouble breathing, snoring, and dry mouth (from mouth breathing).

To wrap this up, I wanted to include a questionnaire made by the Ohio Sleep Medicine Institute that, in my opinion, does a beautifully straightforward job of helping you recognize if you are exhibiting symptoms related to sleep apnea. It's called the STOP-BANG Questionnaire (note the words in all capitals that spell out "stop bang" as a handy acronym). Answer each of the following questions with a yes or no:

1. Do you SNORE loudly (louder than talking or loud enough to be heard through closed doors)?
2. Do you often feel TIRED, fatigued, or sleepy during the daytime?
3. Has anyone OBSERVED you stop breathing during your sleep?
4. Do you have or are you being treated for high blood PRESSURE?
5. Is your BMI more than thirty-five?
6. Is your AGE over fifty years old?
7. Is your NECK circumference greater than sixteen inches?
8. Is your GENDER male?

If you answered yes to two or fewer of these questions, you are at low risk of OSA. With three to four yeses, you are at intermediate risk, and with five to eight, you have a high risk of OSA. If you answered yes to three or more, schedule an appointment with your primary care physician today—*and then maybe go see your dentist!*

As you can see, there aren't any particular bacteria here that are causing the issue—our mouth structure and how it affects the mechanics of our breathing can cause just as many problems as bacteria can. The good news is that structural issues can be discovered and addressed by your dentist. Let's look at some of the awesome ways you and your dentist can help alleviate these apneic symptoms.

FIXING OSA

Probably the go-to solution for OSA that comes up in people's minds is the continuous positive airway pressure device, more commonly known as the CPAP. If you've never seen one of these bad boys, it's a machine that attaches to your face (Ridley Scotts's *Alien*-style) and makes you look and sound like a knockoff Darth Vader. The face mask seals around your nose and/or mouth and provides a constant stream of high-pressured air to keep your airway forced open, thus letting you sleep the night through and sidestepping all that OSA does to your body. Here's the issue: *nobody wants to wear the damn thing.* Studies that measure CPAP compliance (defined as using the therapy for an average of four hours a night for at least 70 percent of nights) show that somewhere between 29 and 83 percent of patients are noncompliant due to removing the device early in the night or not using it altogether.[57] Basically, people are trying to use it but become so flustered that they end up ripping it off after a few hours, and I don't blame them. Imagine someone sticking a rubber hose in your mouth, cranking on an air compressor, and saying, "Sleep tight!" Or even better, think of one of your "late-night escapades" with your partner: "Hey baby, wanna get down?" "Oh yeah! Hang on one sec." *flicks on machine* *BrrrrrUUUUUMMMMMM!* It just isn't natural (or sexy). But a better alternative for many is a mandibular advancement device, or oral appliance. Basically, this little guy looks like a mouthguard on a hinge.

When you order an oral appliance, your dentist will take measurements or molds of your teeth and have it custom-made for you. Once you get it, you just pop it in before bed. While sleeping, the mandibular advancement device will advance your mandible (jawbone), which "lengthens" the mouth. In a nutshell, this device creates a simple movement that accomplishes what those with bruxism are unconsciously doing (jutting their

57 David Repasky, "Why CPAP Compliance Is Important & Tips on Improving Your Therapy," CPAP Blog, May 4, 2023, https://www.cpap.com/blog/cpap-compliance/#:~:text=If%20you%20have%20trouble%20 maintaining,they%20stop%20using%20it%20altogether.

jaw forward and getting their tongue out of the way) to open up the airway and let them breathe—*all without raising the electric bill!*

Unfortunately, most medical insurance requires that a person try the CPAP first. Why? Because insurance companies are about dollars and cents and not health and wellness. To be fair, CPAPs are only required by insurance when someone has *severe* sleep apnea. Those with mild to moderate cases can go straight to an appliance. Once someone with a severe case fails the compliance requirements (which they will because, again, who can get their groove on when looking like Bane from Christopher Nolan's *The Dark Knight Rises*?), they can get an oral appliance. In extreme cases, it's recommended that a person use both devices. This works to aid in their overall comfort because the oral appliance will hold their airway open, which allows for less air pressure to be needed to overcome any obstruction.

A quick note about sleeping pills: there are some patients out there that know they need to sleep and will come to the conclusion to simply pop some trazodone or Ambien (sleeping pills) to keep from waking up. Hopefully, by reading this far, you'll already understand the inherent danger of this—*people with sleep apnea keep waking up because if they don't, they'll die.* When choking in your sleep, your brain jolts you awake to break the REM paralysis so you can breathe again. If you're in a chemically induced state of slumber, your brain can't send the signals it needs to save your life, and then it's lights out for good. Basically, not sleeping isn't the real problem with sleep apnea.

GET YOURSELF TESTED

Surely, by now you have at least an inkling whether or not you or a loved one is suffering from sleep apnea. If you suspect this at all, it's worth it to get yourself tested—it's not as big a deal as you think. Remember when I described the two types of sleep apnea? While central sleep apnea does need to be tested in a hospital, being that it has to do with your brain, obstructive sleep apnea can be tested right at home! Plus, many dentists, like myself, are equipped with the tools and services needed to test for and treat OSA (however, they cannot legally diagnose apnea; only a medical doctor can do that).

The testing equipment includes a little iPad-like device that connects (via Bluetooth) to a few different things. There's a pulse oximeter that goes on your finger, a nasal cannula (the hose that sits just inside both of your nostrils), and a band that goes around your chest. All of this measures your blood oxygen levels, airflow, heart rate, and effort in breathing while you sleep. These metrics are used to determine how many apneic events you have during the night (the standard is when you stop breathing for ten seconds or more and there's a decrease in the oxygen saturation of your blood). This data is then used to calculate your apnea–hypopnea index, or AHI number. In order to receive a diagnosis of sleep apnea, your AHI number must come back as five or more per hour—that is, you need to be almost choking to death every twelve minutes to be considered apneic. And don't forget, some people are having obstructions as many as seventy times per hour. That's more than once a minute! No wonder they can't get any sleep.

If you take the test and it comes back negative, that's great! But you're not in the clear. Remember, our muscles and tissues weaken as we get older, especially in postmenopausal women and those with osteoporosis. This degradation easily leads to obstructions. What I'm trying to say is you need to be conscious of the symptoms of OSA to catch it early, and to be safe, you should take an apnea test every few years or when symptoms arise. If you're young and free of symptoms, you can test yourself every five years. And why wouldn't you? You can test from home!

THE MOUTH-BREATH CONNECTION

Do you know why people spend so much money on the front door of their houses? *Because it's important.* A front door is an entryway to your home; you need something strong that keeps out intruders and something nice that sets the tone of your entire domicile. The mouth is no different. If you take time to work on the "entryway to your body," the rest of your body will fall in line, whether that's stopping bad bacteria or otherwise. Here, we saw how even the structure of the mouth can hamper your breathing and cause serious harm to your overall health. My longtime patient Maria saw exactly that. Her overall health drastically improved by simply adjusting her mouth with an oral appliance, which let her breathe *and just get some sleep.* Without even knowing you, I'm certain the same could be possible for many readers right now.

We're almost done with how oral health impacts your well-being. The last topic to discuss before we go into solutions is oral bacteria's effect on arguably the most important organ in your body: your brain. If you think you'll be using your gray matter in the future, then this is *not* a chapter you want to skip.

CHAPTER 9

Brain Health: Alzheimer's/Dementia

"HIYA, TOOTS!" ETHEL, EVERYONE'S FAVORITE SPUNKY older lady and one of my favorite patients, was in my office first thing in the morning, early as always.

"Hi, Ethel! So nice to see you again. How are you feeling these days?"

"Oh, please," she said, exasperated, waving me off. "Everyone's always asking me 'how I'm doing' as if I'm an old woman or something. I've never been stronger!"

"Fair enough," I chuckled. "What can I do for you today?"

"I need one of those mouth guard appliance what-cha-ma-call-ems."

"A sleep appliance, you mean?"

Ethel snapped her fingers and pointed, "Yep! That's the one!"

"Okay, how come?" I queried.

"Well, I'll tell ya. So you know I have sleep apnea?"

"Yes, I remember. You have a CPAP device."

"I do, but I hate the dern thing—can't sleep with it hugging my face. The doc says I have to wear it because I keep having TIAs at night, but I ain't gonna do it. It's uncomfortable! But he does make a point about me keeping my brain so I came in to see if you'd—"

I interrupted, "Wait a second. Did you say TIAs?"

"Uh-huh."

"TIAs…as in, you're having mini-strokes all throughout the night?"

"Yeah, you got it, hon. So like I was saying, I won't wear it and wanted to see if you'll make me one of those thingies instead; the—what'd you call 'em again?"

Of course I agreed to help, but wow, was my head spinning. This lady just told me how she was having transient ischemic attacks at night as if she were recapping the latest episode of her favorite sitcom. Within a few days, we had the appliance made and sent it to her. Hopefully, Ethel is doing better with the guard in place and *not stroking out in her sleep anymore.*

* * *

The mind is a terrible thing to waste—it's the CPU to our biological machines (our bodies), and when it goes, so do we. If Ethel hadn't done something for her sleep apnea, she would be at serious risk of damaging her brain—losing her memory and developing dementia.

In this chapter, we'll discuss more on the connection between brain health and our mouths, with dementia being one of the side effects when our mouths work against us.

HEALTHY MIND, HEALTHY BODY

Medically, *dementia* is an all-encompassing term that labels the cognitive decline associated with damaged neurons (brain nerves) and their connections in our brains. It's this damage that causes the all-too-familiar symptoms of a failing memory and changes in a personality. Though it's important to note that dementia goes beyond just "having a bad memory"—the brain damage that occurs affects our cognitive function. To understand the difference, compare how fast you can remember something (recall) versus how quickly you can solve a problem (cognitive functions).

Early signs of dementia can include the following examples of cognitive decline:

- Difficulty concentrating
- Memory loss
- Increasing difficulty in carrying out familiar daily tasks (e.g., becoming confused over the correct change when shopping)
- Struggles in following a conversation or finding the right word
- Being confused about the time and/or whereabouts
- Distinct mood changes

Dementia, sadly, ends with complete memory loss and an inability to carry out basic daily functions (e.g., sitting up and eating), leaving a shell of the person who was once full of life. The average age for dementia onset is eighty-three years and it is typically diagnosed *after* ten years of cognitive decline.

THE MAIN TYPES

The three main varieties of dementia are Alzheimer's, vascular dementia, and Parkinson's (I bet you didn't know the last one was a form of dementia).

Alzheimer's, accounting for 70 percent of all dementia cases, is typically acquired from a lifetime neural inflammation, which can be caused by a bacterial infection, poor blood sugar control, or even viruses. However, there are a number of gene mutations that can also lead to an increased risk of early-onset Alzheimer's. Apolipoprotein A (ApoE4) is one of these (it is also the gene affecting heart disease risk).[58]

You see, the brain needs cholesterol; it's what lines our neurons and helps with signaling in the brain. Seventy-five percent of cholesterol is made by the liver, and 25 percent comes from food, but regardless of where it comes from, the brain is responsible for most of its own cholesterol production and keeps it local with the use of the blood-brain barrier. The blood-brain barrier can be broken down by stress, inflammation, diseases, smoking, and having the ApoE4 mutation. A leaky blood-brain barrier disrupts the brain's ability to protect its local cholesterol and can lead to neurodegenerative diseases. Further, in people with ApoE4 gene mutations, the cholesterol balance and lipid metabolism in the brain is disrupted, leading to the formation of triglycerides, which damages our neurons, leading to Alzheimer's. And this is not uncommon; approximately 25 percent of the population has this mutation. Luckily, gene tests are available, and I highly recommend you take one. This is not something you want to wait and catch after it starts.

Having one ApoE4 mutation increases Alzheimer's risk by two to three times. Having both genes mutated increases the risk eight to twelve times. But remember, we are not our genes. There are things you can do to mitigate your risk! We will discuss these later in the book.

---

58   "Do You Have the Heart Attack Gene?" BaleDoneen Method, accessed May 19, 2023, https://baledoneen. com/blog/do-you-have-the-heart-attack-gene/#.

The hallmark of Alzheimer's disease is the buildup of beta-amyloid and tau proteins around nerve cells in the brain causing the brain to shrink and the neurotransmitters to malfunction.

Taking choline supplements to prevent Alzheimer's looks promising for people with the ApoE4 gene mutation.

Vascular dementia is the medical term for what Ethel was at risk of developing because her sleep apnea at night led to transient ischemic attacks (TIAs), or mini-strokes. Vascular dementia is often caused by a reduction of blood flow to the brain, usually from obstructive sleep apnea, chronic inflammation of blood vessels, smoking, high blood pressure, being overweight, and having diabetes (dementia is often considered the "diabetes of the brain"). In particular, these patients may experience more problem-solving issues over general memory loss.

The final major type of dementia is a result of Parkinson's disease. Scientists are still unsure what causes it, but whatever the origin, Parkinson's disease occurs when the nerve cells become damaged or die off, which decreases dopamine in the brain (dopamine smooths our muscle functions). A classic symptom of Parkinson's is seeing someone with the shakes (and no, it's not from drinking too many martinis the night before). Due to their poor motor function, Parkinson's patients often also develop poorer and poorer oral hygiene as the disease develops, which further exacerbates the issue as oral bacteria causes neural inflammation (the same can be said for all types of dementia due to general cognitive decline).

A CLOSER LOOK AT ALZHEIMER'S

Because Alzheimer's is such a large part of the total number of dementia cases, I want to spend a little more time with it.

Alzheimer's affects 14 percent of the population (one in seven people), and women are twice as likely as men to develop Alzheimer's. Why? Possibly because they tend to live longer, but also possibly because of the reduction of estrogen after menopause. Estrogen has a vital role in memory and in ensuring neurotransmitters in the brain function properly. Additionally, women are usually the caregivers; thus they tend to have more stress, which drives disease in general and is believed to play a role in Alzheimer's.[59]

Our brain is protected by the blood-brain barrier—its job is to keep out anything that can damage the brain. It's a bit like McAfee virus protection on your computer. The software keeps out viruses that can harm and shut down your computer. But when the software gets penetrated or overridden, you can have a complete system failure.

So what's the mouth got to do with Alzheimer's disease? Well, Pg has been found in the brains of patients who had Alzheimer's, which leads researchers to believe that in some cases, Alzheimer's can be the result of a chronic bacterial invasion that triggered neural inflammation. Pg also releases a toxic protein called gingipains, which inhibits proper Tau protein function, something necessary for normal neuron function. The end result of Pg infection is the formation of beta-amyloid plaques. The thought that plaques are formed to protect the neurons from a bacterial invasion is spawning much research

[59] Nicholas J. Justice, "The Relationship between Stress and Alzheimer's Disease," *Neurobiology of Stress* 8 (February 2018): 127–133, https://doi.org/10.1016/j.ynstr.2018.04.002.

and interest in possibly identifying a bacterial infection as a direct cause of Alzheimer's.[60]

Researchers are finding Pg in cerebrospinal fluid of patients with Alzheimer's disease, which could lead to testing for it and diagnosis in living patients.[61]

It all works like this: when bacteria cross the BBB (blood-brain barrier), our bodies freak out, and rightly so. Our BBB should be impenetrable to bacteria, viruses, fungi, and so on, but it lets in glucose so our brain can function properly. When a patient suffers from chronic inflammation (from an oral infection, for example), the BBB breaks down and no longer works properly, and then bacteria can enter the brain. In an attempt to save itself, our body will wrap beta-amyloid proteins around our neurons to protect them from the invading bacteria. This works much like a sheath, or how the roof closes over a sports arena when it rains. The amyloid proteins work perfectly in protecting the neurons. However, this leads to a toxic change in Tau proteins. It is believed that Tau proteins work together to starve the neurons from receiving nutrients; they "choke" the neurons, eventually killing them. This causes inflammation in the brain as well as causing the brain to shrink, which leads to cognitive symptoms that we see on the outside. Effectively, the body kills the brain to save itself.

Alzheimer's is only able to be confirmed after death with an

---

60 Stephen S. Dominy et al., "*Porphyromonas gingivalis* in Alzheimer's Disease Brains: Evidence for Disease Causation and Treatment with Small-Molecule Inhibitors," *Science Advances* 5, no. 1 (January 2019): eaau3333, https://doi.org/10.1126/sciadv.aau3333.

61 Debora Mackenzie, "We May Finally Know What Causes Alzheimer's—And How to Stop It," New Scientist, last updated January 30, 2019, https://www.newscientist.com/article/2191814-we-may-finally-know-what-causes-alzheimers-and-how-to-stop-it/.

autopsy when the beta-amyloid plaques and brain shrinkage are confirmed ('cause you can't just go hacking around in someone's brain). And for the time being, there is no cure for the disease or way to reverse the damage, only medications to slow the progression and manage the symptoms—when it comes to the brain, once it's done, it's done.

The thing is, research is changing so rapidly that this book will probably be outdated on this subject by the time of its release. In fact, at the time of this writing, new research is confirming beta-amyloid proteins are still the issue with Alzheimer's, but is also noticing and looking at the loss of normal, soluble beta-amyloid proteins instead of beta-amyloid plaque accumulation.[62] Regardless, an infection causing the changes is still a concern.

WHAT ISN'T DEMENTIA?

You might be able to tell that the medical community has trouble identifying dementia—it's true; such is the nature of the brain. As mentioned before, an ironclad diagnosis is unavailable until postmortem, but there are plenty of ways to get close, namely with psychological exams. There's a big difference between just losing something and being frustrated versus becoming stressed, confused, and the search ending with you not knowing what you were doing in the first place. If you are concerned you or a loved one is developing Alzheimer's or dementia, go to alz.org to take a quick test.

---

62 Andrea Sturchio et al., "High Soluble Amyloid-ß42 Predicts Normal Cognition in Amyloid-Positive Individuals with Alzheimer's Disease-Causing Mutations," *Journal of Alzheimer's Disease* 90, no. 1 (2022): 333–348, https://doi.org/10.3233/JAD-220808.

THE ROOT CAUSES OF DEMENTIA

People tend to associate dementia with old age, which is often the case. But remember, dementia is more than memory loss—it's actual brain damage, meaning dementia can develop in anyone. The preventable leading cause of Alzheimer's is poor blood sugar control (another reason Alzheimer's is called "the diabetes of the brain"). The other leading preventable cause is basically just "stuff getting in the brain." For example, the bacterium that the body is responding to with the beta-amyloid proteins is one of those we've been becoming familiar with: Pg.

Pg was one of the few known bacteria that are able to cross the blood-brain barrier, and Alzheimer's patients are found to specifically have Pg infections in the brain. *Coincidence? I think not.* Also, recent studies are showing that Fn can also cross the blood-brain barrier and, while not the cause of Alzheimer's, is able to accelerate the disease by encouraging inflammation in the brain.[63] The science here is constantly changing, but the trend seems to be discovering that "stuff" getting into the brain is a root cause of Alzheimer's.

Another major "mind invader" is HSV, or herpes. Now you might be thinking, "What on earth does herpes have to do with dementia? Dr. Lee, are you having any of the six warning signs listed above?" Well, herpes has more to do with the brain than you think—and by the way, the answer is no. I feel great! Ninety percent of all adults have had HSV at some point in their lives, whether it was a cold sore, chicken pox, shingles, or whatever. However, a sign of the ApoE4 gene mutation is recurring cold sores after a herpes infection. If you have both the mutation

---

63   Hongle Wu et al., "The Periodontal Pathogen *Fusobacterium nucleatum* Exacerbates Alzheimer's Pathogenesis via Specific Pathways," *Frontiers in Aging Neuroscience* 14 (2022), https://doi.org/10.3389/fnagi.2022.912709.

and have ever contracted HSV, your risk of developing dementia goes up by 60 percent! How can this be? I'll explain.

It all has to do with the type 1 form of HSV—a.k.a. "the kissing disease"—which is often contracted when an individual is a child. (I'm not going to discuss type 2 HSV, which is the genital disease. You'll need a different doctor for that!)

When you contract "the kissing disease" as a child, you experience such symptoms as fever, swollen lymph nodes, and mouth sores, all of which usually resolve within two weeks, never to be seen again. However, when those of us with the ApoE4 gene mutation contract the virus, it enters our brain (remember how ApoE4 affects the BBB?) and then remains dormant for years. Whenever peripheral infections occur in the body, such as with COVID-19 or anything we've discussed so far, HSV is reactivated and creates neuroinflammation in the brain, thus producing dementia.[64] Pretty wild, huh?

If you have recurring cold sores, talk to your dentist about them! They can prescribe acyclovir, a medication that can be taken regularly or when you feel the tingle at the beginning of an outbreak. Dentists can also use lasers over a cold sore when it is just beginning to prevent the outbreak.

It's important to note that none of this actually *causes* dementia but only accelerates and/or increases the risk of the

64 "More recently, a study by Bae et al. using National Health Insurance Service data in Korea analyzed 229,594 individuals aged ≥ 50 years. Patients with HZ had a higher risk of dementia (adjusted HR, 1.12, 95% CI, 1.05–1.19). Of the 34,505 patients with HZ, 28,873 (84%) had received antiviral treatment (acyclovir, famciclovir, or valaciclovir). The treated group showed a significantly lower risk of dementia (HR 0.76, 95% CI, 0.65–0.90)." Ruth F. Itzhaki, "Overwhelming Evidence for a Major Role for Herpes Simplex Virus Type 1 (HSV1) in Alzheimer's Disease (AD); Underwhelming Evidence Against," Vaccines 9, no. 6 (2021): 679, https://doi.org/10.3390/vaccines9060679.

disease—we still aren't completely sure what causes it, exactly, but I digress. The last major "thing" that gets in the brain is the fungus *Candida albicans*, better known in the mouth as thrush. But I don't want to talk about that just yet as it *majorly* has to do with oral health.

FROM THE BRAIN TO THE MOUTH (OR VICE VERSA)

Speaking of oral health, let's dive into how your mouth affects brain health. For starters, the obvious connection is through Pg and Fn. In fact, a recent study has shown that deaths caused by and diagnoses of Alzheimer's in patients sixty-five and older were associated with antibodies of oral Pg as well as the presence of periodontal disease before dementia.[65] Or, as Anne O. Rice, a specialist on periodontal inflammation says, "Oral inflammation triggers neural inflammation."[66]

However, the real connection to the mouth is in the compounding effect that poor oral hygiene has on dementia. You see, not only do oral infections spread to the rest of the body, eventually leading to the brain, but the deterioration and tooth loss derived from gum disease creates poor chewing ability that leads to nutritional deficiencies, which aid the progression of dementia. This, in turn, creates greater cognitive decline, which exacerbates all of the aforementioned complications—the cycle continues. It's very possible that dementia both begins and ends in the mouth.

Some of my more sleuthy readers will have already made the

65 May A. Beydoun et al., "Clinical and Bacterial Markers of Periodontitis and Their Association with Incident All-Cause and Alzheimer's Disease Dementia in a Large National Survey," *Journal of Alzheimer's Disease* 75, no. 1 (2020): 157–172, https://doi.org/10.3233/JAD-200064.

66 Anne O. Rice, "Alzheimer's Disease and Oral-Systemic Health: Bidirectional Care Integration Improving Outcomes," *Frontiers in Oral Health* 2 (2021): 674329, https://doi.org/10.3389/froh.2021.674329.

connection between blood glucose control, dementia, and what I spoke about on how oral bacteria can upset that process. This hunch holds water, as patients with periodontal disease are 2.6 times more likely to develop dementia.[67] Oral bacterial infections, via MMP-8, can create the systemic inflammation that hampers glycemic regulation, which, again, is the number one preventable cause of Alzheimer's. As a patient's cognitive ability declines, so does their oral hygiene, causing *more* bacteria to invade, which progresses dementia even further, and so on and so on…Now we have compounding effects atop compounding effects. Starting to get the picture?

WHY THE ELDERLY?

One of the reasons most dementia patients are primarily older adults isn't just because "old people forget stuff" (remember, we're talking about *cognitive decline* here). It's for two reasons. First, statistically speaking, the older someone is, the more likely they are to have an oral disease, which we now know is directly related to dementia. The second reason is because the elderly are the most likely to be missing teeth, whether that be from prolonged gum disease, cavities or infections, or just having lived longer and experienced more accidents and wear and tear. Researchers have found that adults with missing teeth are 48 percent more likely to develop cognitive impairment and 28 percent more likely to develop dementia, with each missing tooth adding 1.4 percent to the risk of cognitive impairment and 1.1 percent to the risk of dementia.[68] Those missing twenty or

67 Kiyotaro Kondo, Minehisa Niino, and Koichi Shido, "A Case-Control Study of Alzheimer's Disease in Japan—Significance of Life-Styles," *Dementia* 5 (1994): 314–326, https://doi.org/10.1159/000106741.

68 Xiang Qi et al., "Dose-Response Meta-Analysis on Tooth Loss with the Risk of Cognitive Impairment and Dementia," *JAMDA* 22, no. 10 (October 2021): 2039–2045, https://doi.org/10.1016/j.jamda.2021.05.009.

more teeth had a 31 percent higher risk of cognitive impairment, and those with no teeth at all had a 54 percent higher risk of cognitive impairment and a 40 percent higher risk of dementia. This association is largely attributed to these folk being unable to chew up healthy foods, leading them to turn to the easy, high-carb processed snacks instead that are easier to swallow whole and digest versus fibrous fruits and veggies. This leads to a spike in blood sugar and neural inflammation.

Interestingly, researchers also found that if patients had their teeth replaced with implants or dentures, their risk of dementia went back to levels of those who had retained their teeth. Sounds great, right? Well, maybe not. Being that dementia is irreversible, once a dementia patient receives their dentures, they either forget to wear them or lose their ability to tolerate them, leading to the nutritional deficiencies and compounding effects mentioned above. But the real complication with dentures and dementia comes from how the porous nature of their acrylic makeup is the perfect breeding ground for *Candida albicans* (thrush). This yeast is a naturally occurring fungus that occurs on and in the body, but if it makes it deep inside (like through the mouth), big problems occur. Candida is always present in the mouth, but a healthy microbiome keeps it at bay. However, in the case of denture wearers, they often are on medications that exacerbate dry mouth, or they sleep with their dentures and forget to clean them. This, in addition to the denture pores, makes a perfect environment for thrush to thrive.

Yeast is another substance that can cross the BBB and, like HSV, is toxic and causes neuroinflammation. When this happens, immune cells in our brain activate and secrete molecules that trap the yeast inside cells. These cell-trapped fungi group together to create induced glial granulomas, or "figs," inside the brain (similar to the beta-amyloid proteins). This creates, you guessed it again, *more* cognitive decline, which causes patients to clean their dentures even less often, which creates more yeast. Basically, when dementia patients don't wear their dentures, they eat poorly—which causes inflammation—and when they do wear them, they get a yeast infection. Like I often say, "Dentures cause dementia."

Antibiotics can be a double-edged sword. While they may be necessary to fight off a lingering, severe infection, they are not very selective and can kill off our healthy microbiome, and thrush can take over. When people take antibiotics for a sinus infection, they are often left with yeast in the sinuses, which has just a short distance to travel before it gets to the brain.

I'm not saying antibiotics are evil and to never take them. Just don't pop them like candy, especially for a viral infection like a cold or the flu.

PREVENTION

The good news is that one-third of all Alzheimer's cases are preventable.[69] Many of the methods to prevent cognitive decline can be accomplished via oral care, whether at home or by your dentist—the easiest of which is just brushing your teeth or helping an elderly parent, for example, brush theirs. This simple act will knock back the amount of would-be blood-surfing bad bacteria in your mouth (Pg and Fn in this case). Brushing, flossing, and using mouthwash are kind of the "just diet and exercise" approach of the dental world; you can't go wrong with these. Not to mention the clear connection of oral care to tooth retention and tooth retention to the lower risk of dementia.

Something else you can do is encourage them to get any lost

---

69   Rice, "Alzheimer's Disease and Oral-Systemic Health."

teeth replaced. We need homeostasis in our mouths, meaning they need to be balanced—that's why your teeth are paired. For each bottom tooth, you should have a top tooth. We also need balance from side to side; you can't expect only half your teeth to do the job of a full set.

All that is to say, any tooth that gets removed needs to be replaced. Think about it: what other body part do you not want to replace if you lose it? It's important for their self-esteem, for systemic health and nutritional status, and for aging!

THE MOUTH-DEMENTIA CONNECTION

The mind and the mouth are more connected than you might have thought, but hey, they are only a few inches away from one another. Just as we've seen with the other ailments, when oral bacteria aren't dealt with, they disrupt health on a systemic level, this time leading to one of the most devastating diseases a person can have. Aside from the bacterial connection, the fact that Ethel wasn't getting the quality sleep she needed also put her at risk of damaging her brain with a stroke. Ethel was right to heed her doctor's advice on "keeping her brain" lest she become only a husk of the upbeat lady whom I've known. And fortunately, CPAP machines and oral appliances from your dentist can course-correct damage to the brain for short-term memory.

I have seen firsthand in many patients how losing your teeth can put you in the grave expeditiously. Now, I advise my elderly patients to keep their teeth at all costs. "You have lived your entire life and worked hard so you could coast through your twilight years. You deserve this," I tell them.

If you want to live a long and healthy life, mind your teeth! I know: I'm a dentist, and of course I'd say that. But there is a direct correlation between the number of teeth you retain and the average number of years lived. Studies *clearly* show a 4 percent increase in the five-year survival rate per additional tooth retained at the age of seventy. The tipping point for survival is keeping at least twenty teeth.[70] Additionally, many elderly view tooth loss as a loss in the quality of life; no longer can they or do they desire to socialize, have dinners, play instruments, sing, or do other enjoyable activities, which can lead to depression—meaning that not only do you have a shorter life when you lose teeth, but also it may not be the life you'd want to live.

If you lose your hearing or vision, sever a limb, or one of your organ functions stops, you're considered to have a disability. We need to start thinking of losing teeth in the same way. If what I was writing in this book were common knowledge, masticatory disabilities would be commonplace, and help would be readily available. I suppose I'm trying to start that movement. Remember, all the horribleness of what I've been showing you *doesn't have to happen*. The helpful tools *are* there. The resources *are* available. We just need to have the awareness that good oral health means good system health.

So, with that said, let's look at what you and your dentist can *do* to help you live a long and healthy life with a mouth full of teeth. It's time for action!

---

70 Toshinobu Hirotomi et al., "Number of Teeth and 5-Year Mortality in an Elderly Population," *Community Dentistry and Oral Epidemiology* 43, no. 3 (January 2015): 226–231, https://doi.org/10.1111/cdoe.12146.

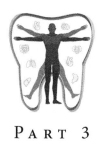

PART 3

THE SOLUTIONS!

CHAPTER 10

Change Your Mouth— Change Your Life

THANK YOU FOR STAYING WITH ME HERE! I REALIZE I might have scared the hell out of you with all that talk about what could go wrong in your mouth. Please know I'm not fear-mongering. On an almost-daily basis (and it would be daily if we were open on Sundays), people show up in the chairs at my practice with troubled mouths. The good news, which is something I hope you also gleaned from the preceding chapters, is that there are plenty of things you can do, and that your dentist can do, to clean up your mouth and heal what's going on in there, which will help the rest of your body too.

In other words, you don't have to use your mouth as the beginning point of a downward spiral into poor health. You can use it as something that will elevate your health and well-being. You've just gotta make some lifestyle changes if you want that to happen.

There are no "get out of jail free" cards here, no hall passes from your dentist. It's time to pretend you're an adult until it becomes habitual and do all those things you know you're supposed to do but never quite got around to starting, beginning with brushing.

THE OLDEST ADVICE IN THE DENTAL WORLD

"Did you brush your teeth?"

"Yes, Mom…"

"Open up. Lemme see."

Since our first tooth broke in when we were infants, we've all been told good brushing matters. And despite growing up with adults constantly reiterating the need for it, not all of us are good brushers on a consistent basis. There are so many reasons why: we get home so late at night, and we're exhausted; we're camping and forgot to pack a brush, so we use a finger… actually, I'm not sure what the reasons are. I'm a busy person with an active life outside of work, and I still brush my teeth a couple of times a day.

I think many people have the mentality that if they can't see something happening right now, then it isn't happening. That's why smokers continue to smoke—they don't see the evidence of cancer in their lungs as soon as they snuff out a cigarette, so it's hard for them to believe it will ever be a problem. Yes, I just compared the dangers of not brushing your teeth with those of smoking cigarettes. If you think I'm speaking in hyperbole here, then reread the last nine chapters before continuing.

BRUSH LIKE YOU MEAN IT!

Brushing is just the beginning. Let's look at the right way to do all those things you tell your dentist you do oh so well. Which, by the way, we know you're lying about.

Brushing

I always recommend using an electric toothbrush—the kind that plugs into a wall, not the battery-operated type. A typical electric toothbrush will brush teeth at speeds between 2,500 and 7,500 strokes per minute. Given that you manually brush at 300 strokes per minute (probably fewer than that when you're brushing before dawn), it's easy to see how much more an electric brush can give you during your two minutes. And you are brushing for two minutes, right? Thirty seconds on each quadrant? Another benefit of electric toothbrushes is that they often have timers, so you're not mentally counting *one Mississippi, two Mississippi*...I like to put mine on "deep clean" or "gum therapy," which gives me three minutes of total brushing time. If you have gum problems or are prone to inflammation, I highly suggest you do this!

You know this, but I'm going to say it anyway: brush at least twice a day, and replace your toothbrush (or brush head, if electric) every three months or after you've been sick. Be picky about where you keep your brush. If your spouse or partner has gum disease, don't put yours so close that the bristles can touch. Never use those communal toothbrush cups with holes close to each other for manual toothbrushes. That's just disgusting. And for heaven's sake, do not store your toothbrush next to your toilet!

One final note on brushing: it is possible to kill your gums with kindness, meaning you can brush them so hard that you brush them away. Make sure your brush has soft or ultrasoft bristles. The medium/hard ones are too strong for gum tissue and may cause recession and sensitivity.

And to make your brushing really count, you gotta use the right toothpaste.

One thing to ask regarding your toothpaste is "What kind of chemicals are in my products?" Some chemicals in toothpaste can be irritating to your gums. They also strip away the lining of your mouth and may cause canker sores. Sodium lauryl sulfate (SLS) is such a chemical. It's often added as a foaming agent because some people have a hard time believing anything is getting clean unless there are a bunch of bubbles involved. Then I have patients come in and tell me they think they're allergic to their toothpaste because their mouth is reacting to the foaming agent. SLS is also used as an insecticide! Last I checked, I did not have any mosquitos in my mouth.

Another harmful chemical is titanium dioxide. It's a chemical that makes our toothpaste white. It literally has zero health benefits; it is just a colorant. Meanwhile, many studies suggest it is carcinogenic and causes organ toxicity.[71]

Other chemicals are just bad for you, like the antimicrobials that are in some toothpaste. Why would you want to kill the good bacteria on your teeth? You don't. But antimicrobials don't have the ability to distinguish between good and bad bacteria.

Triclosan is an antibacterial agent that was used in soap and toothpaste. It was taken off the market in 2018 when it was found to cause colitis and colon cancer in mice. Then, in 2019, the ADA discovered it caused osteoporosis and negatively impacted thyroid hormone production. Its use is banned in bodywashes and soaps but is still allowed in toothpaste! Read the labels! You just don't know what you don't know!

Fluoride is another common additive to toothpaste because it does help fight cavities. Before the anti-fluoride crowd starts rappelling through the windows, note that I'm going to give

---

71   Matej Skocaj et al., "Titanium Dioxide in Our Everyday Life; Is It Safe?" *Radiology and Oncology* 45, no. 4 (December 2011): 227–247, https://doi.org/10.2478/v10019-011-0037-0.

some fluoride-free alternatives in a bit. But the reason that fluoride is used in the dental field so widely is that it does some amazing things for your mouth and teeth—it just needs to be used in the correct situation, and not everyone needs it.

Fluoride works in two different ways. In the first, when the pH in a mouth drops below 5.5, minerals start to dissolve out of teeth, the initial stage of cavity formation. When that happens, fluoride will combine with hydroxyapatite (another tooth mineral) to form something called fluorapatite, which gets deposited back into the tooth. So in this first way, fluoride works to remineralize teeth.

The second way it works is that because fluorapatite is more resistant to acidic pH, it will not dissolve until the pH drops below 4.5. So in this way, it strengthens the teeth.

Because of the effects of fluoride, some municipalities began adding it to their water supply back in the second half of the twentieth century. They did it because dental decay is the most prevalent disease in children in the United States—at one time it was the leading cause of children missing school. According to the CDC, following the introduction of fluoridated water and the addition of fluoride to toothpaste and other dental products, the average number of missing or decaying teeth in twelve-year-old children dropped by 68 percent between the late 1960s and early 1990s.[72] There are some countries that do not allow fluoride in their water supply, and their cavity rate is low, so it is multifactorial. And it is true that fluoride is a neurotoxin when ingested at high levels (is the government trying to poison us?!).

However, while effective, fluoride does need to be used in small amounts and in appropriate situations—for example,

---

72 Centers for Disease Control and Prevention, "Achievements in Public Health 1900–1999: Fluoridation of Drinking Water to Prevent Dental Caries," *Morbidity and Mortality Weekly Report* 48, no. 41 (October 1999): 933–940, https://www.cdc.gov/mmwr/preview/mmwrhtml/mm4841a1.htm.

when patients have a history of cavities. If they use the right amount and they do not swallow it, fluoride could be of benefit to them. But if someone has never had a cavity before, they don't guzzle soda or sugary drinks, and they have a good diet, then they probably don't need fluoride.

And for those who are fluoride-averse (which is fine to be!), there's nano-hydroxyapatite. It is so safe and effective that, instead of fluoride, hydroxyapatite has been the gold standard in Canada and Japan for decades. Created by NASA in 1970, it is made up of calcium and phosphate and was invented to help restore any bone or tooth loss that astronauts might experience after living in a gravity-free environment during space missions.[73]

Fluoride-free toothpaste alternatives that I recommend include:

- Boka, which is what I personally use
- Nano-hydroxyapatite (N-Ha) toothpaste; our teeth are made up of N-Ha, and this toothpaste puts this mineral back into your teeth
- MI Paste: fluoride-free options available

Brushing is absolutely incredible; such a simple action disrupts bacteria's slimy, filth-ridden world. To be clear, the good bacteria in your mouth also create their own biofilm, but shortly after eating, bad bacteria start to stick to the "healthy plaque," thus making it more pathologic over time. But with brushing, you are continually breaking up the bad biofilm and—hopefully—spitting most of it out. There is one downside to brushing, though, and it's the obvious one: brushing only cleans

---

73 NASA, "Bones in Space," August 19, 2004, https://www.nasa.gov/audience/forstudents/postsecondary/features/F_Bones_in_Space.html.

the tops, fronts, and backs of your teeth—*you still need to clean in between*. So at the risk of sounding like every dentist who ever lived, you need to brush *and* floss.

Get Stringy with It

Everyone tells their dentist they floss every day.

Here's a secret: we can easily tell they're lying.

Yes, you need to floss every day! Twice, in fact. There's no Big Floss conspiracy out there—sorry Facebook. Think about it; you have five surfaces of each tooth: front, back, bottom (or top), left, and right. Brushing only can get to three of those, which leaves 40 percent of your teeth *untouched*! Flossing is the gold standard if you want a healthy mouth.

There's an old dental saying: only floss the teeth you want to keep!

The best way to floss is the way you were taught way back in primary school: pull off a super long piece of floss, wrap it around your fingers, and swipe it between your teeth, making a C-shaped curve around the tooth. Scrape the teeth on either side of the floss five times with this C shape. Pull the floss out and wrap to a clean section. It's not a matter of snapping the floss down hard between your teeth to make your gums bleed and tugging it back out.

A key thing to remember is never to use the same section of the floss twice; keep unwrapping and wrapping as necessary between teeth; otherwise, you'll just deposit the crap you cleaned out from one place into another. You'll know you did a good job if it takes you three to five minutes to complete your mouth.

If flossing is not an option for you (and that doesn't mean because you have to get up five minutes earlier in the morning—I do it every day too!), try using a water pick. The only people who get a hall pass for not flossing are those whose teeth are crammed together so tightly it's impossible to get the floss between them and people who have dexterity issues, like those with arthritis or Parkinson's disease. For them, a water pick will help flush out bacteria that might be stuck between their teeth. (Of course, if you want to be an all-star, water pick and floss every day!) To make the water pick even more effective, put a probiotic mouthwash inside it, mixed with water.

The least effective tool for cleaning between your teeth is a floss pick. These are fine to keep in your pocket or purse to use when you're out someplace and want to remove something that's wedged between your teeth, but they will only move bacteria around your mouth if you use them in more than one place. It's like cleaning your counter with a dirty rag. Why would you do that?

And when you're done, rinse out your mouth.

Rinse and Repeat

While brushing and flossing will break up the biofilm, and you may have spit some of it out, there will probably be some left floating around your mouth. That's why mouthwash is important.

I know what you're thinking here: "Dr. Lee, you just talked about the good bacteria in our mouths. Won't swishing with mouthwash wipe out all oral bacteria?" That's an excellent point, which is why you need to be selective in the products you use. And if you're one of those people who are obsessed with sterilizing your mouth, *STOP.*

You need good bacteria as much as you don't need the bad. That said, we want to stay away from antimicrobial and alcohol-based mouthwashes, which are nonselective in their bacterial destruction (that, and they also dry out your mouth). So let's drop the "the burn says it's working" mentality crap. After all, if your skin were burning, wouldn't you be concerned?

In addition, good bacteria are easier to kill than bad (which explains why infections are hard to get rid of). So if you're using a mouthwash that claims to wipe out 99.99 percent of everything, do you think that the last 0.01 percent that survives is the good or bad kind of bacteria? Yeah, *it's the bad kind*. Survival of the fittest tells us that that remnant of bacteria is the toughest, meanest SOB in your mouth. Why leave it in there?

Let me be clear: my efforts here aren't to say that the big oral health companies are bad. I'm just trying to correct the belief people have of "if I want a healthier mouth, I need to clean *harder*" (read that in a Schwarzenegger voice). Some people are gung-ho and want to annihilate the problem. Yes, take your oral health seriously, but hey, be kind to your body too, okay?

Remember, the point is about balance. Our body, like our mouth, is an ecosystem: a mixture of human genes, cells, and microbes, both good and bad (but we definitely want more good than bad!). If any one thing becomes lopsided, the whole environment will suffer. If this happens in the mouth, as we have been discussing, the oral issue will lead to other issues throughout the body. Just think, 80 percent of our immune cells are in our gut, and nothing gets to our gut except through our mouths. Research shows that one milliliter of saliva contains about 100 million microbes, meaning it's estimated that humans swallow up to 100 billion microbes of bacteria every twenty-four hours. So let's focus on balance so that we get the good microbes in our guts by getting our mouths to work for us.

Hopefully, I haven't scared you off mouthwash. Do know it's important! It will loosen food particles, disrupt the plaque biofilm, and help clean areas of the mouth where you didn't get with your brush.

Look for mouthwashes that are alkaline (that have a high pH), organic, and chemical free. I recommend staying away from any with essential oils as they can disrupt the microbiome and affect the bonding strength of any restorations in your mouth (things like fillings and crowns).

My favorites are:

- Tom's
- Hello products
- CloSYS
- P2 products
- Dr. Brite
- Dental Herb Company
- Invivo Bio.Me Oral is probably my favorite as it's a probiotic mouthwash that boosts my oral immunity.

Keep in mind that I am not paid to recommend any of these products. This is all strictly from my personal experience.

I often get asked about oil pulling. Oil pulling is a safe and effective way to target bad bacteria in your mouth. I advise my patients to see their dentist first and get cleaned up, and then they can maintain at home with oil pulling. I recommend coconut oil as it is antiviral and antibacterial. It also helps support the healthy microbiome in the mouth and is full of healthy fats, which is great for the saliva pellicle.

For oil pulling to be effective, you must hold the oil in your mouth for five minutes before spitting it out. This is an exceptionally long time (especially when I cannot get patients to brush for two minutes), which is why it does not work for most people. Also, if you have extensive dental work in your mouth, I would advise against oil pulling as it could damage your restorations. Use the other options mentioned above.

I don't care what order you brush, floss, and rinse. Just do them all!

There are a few more steps to take if you really want to get an A+ in oral healthcare. They include mouth sprays and tongue scraping.

Mouth Spray

I'm not talking about breath sprays here—steer clear of anything made to cover up the smell of bad breath. They usually contain alcohol, which will dry out your mouth, and don't make me lecture you about xerostomia. And if you have bad breath, that means there is a problem going on; don't cover it up. Go get it checked.

What I'm talking about is using a mouth spray that will help keep your mouth moist as well as neutralize your pH between meals. These are not meant to cover up bad breath but to neutralize your saliva. This isn't a "have to" for good oral health, but a sugar-free one is a handy thing to keep in your pocket or purse to use between meals, particularly ones with acidic foods or drinks.

If you want to give them a try, I recommend:

- Luvbiotics
- CloSYS
- Uncle Harry's

Tongue Scraping

Get ready for something kind of gross to think about: your tongue harbors bacteria. Your tastebuds—all those little bumps on your tongue—provide perfect hiding places for microscopic things like bacteria to set up home. So, while you're brushing your pearly whites to take care of your teeth and gums, baddies from the bacterial world are living it up on your tongue.

Bacteria on the tongue can lead to bad breath, which is bad enough. But to make matters worse, the bacteria don't stay there. They surf on your saliva to reach your teeth, where they cause cavities, and your gums, where they can lead to periodontal disease. So you really do want to pay attention to your tongue and clean it.

The best way to clear the bacteria from your tongue is by using a tongue scraper. These are metal tools with a U-shape on one end that you run across the surface of your tongue. If you've never done that before, be prepared: removing that coating off your tongue could get ugly, especially if you have acid reflux or were sick enough to be vomiting recently.

If you don't have a tongue scraper now, but the above paragraph made you just order one off of Amazon, you can use your toothbrush to scrub your tongue until it arrives. It will remove some of the bacteria, but it's not as effective as tongue scraping. In fact, a study from 2004 found tongue scraping to remove 30 percent more sulfur compounds (the stuff that makes you stink) than using a soft-bristle brush.[74] Sulfur compounds are what make bad breath, in case you're wondering.

If you're still not convinced tongue scraping is worth the effort, there is an added benefit from doing it: better-tasting

---

74   Vinícius Pedrazzi et al., "Tongue-Cleaning Methods: A Comparative Clinical Trial Employing a Toothbrush and a Tongue Scraper," *Journal of Periodontology* 75, no. 7 (July 2004): 1009–1012, https://doi.org/10.1902/jop.2004.75.7.1009.

food! Many people discover they can taste their foods better after they've started scraping their tongues on a regular basis. So it's very possible that having a clean mouth will help you enjoy all those vegetables you should be eating but just don't like. Who knows? Maybe you'll even discover a penchant for Brussels sprouts. Which would be a good thing, because part of developing your own personalized wellness plan (as you'll soon see) is incorporating a well-balanced diet with foods that will keep your mouth (and the rest of your body) healthy.

But, if you're still not convinced tongue scraping provides any benefit, then I challenge you to Google "hairy tongue."

When you're done, let's talk a little about why these oral habits are good ones: they get rid of unwanted guests.

PLAQUE AND TARTAR—UNWELCOME GUESTS WHO NEVER WANT TO LEAVE

Brushing isn't just repeating doctor-recommended rhetoric. It sets the very foundation of oral hygiene by removing bacteria-filled plaque. Let's talk about tooth plaque for a minute; it's something you've probably heard of. But do you know what it actually is? The most common answer I get to that question is plaque is left-behind food. *buzzer sound* Sorry, wrong answer. Remember when you noticed you had spinach stuck on one of your front teeth only after flirting with someone? *That* was left-behind food.

While it's related to food, plaque is something altogether quite different. Take your fingernail and scratch your tooth. See the gooey white stuff under your nails? That's plaque. (If you didn't get any, scratch a little harder. If your nail is still clean, congratulations! You're doing a good job of cleaning *that* part of *that* tooth. How are the rest of your teeth measuring up?)

The makeup of that off-white goo is bad bacteria and the

excrement they made from digesting the food you just ate. Yep, you've got bacteria shit under your nails now. Go wash your hands; I'll wait here.

When bacteria and bacteria poo build up enough to create plaque, they form a biofilm on your tooth surface, which makes your teeth even stickier, so they attract even more microscopic friends. This is how bacteria will colonize your mouth—they set up the perfect environment for themselves to live, work, and play on your teeth. But they live like bad citizens who destroy their planet while inhabiting it.

Within forty-eight hours, that biofilm, if left alone, will react with the minerals in your saliva to calcify (harden with calcium) and turn into tartar (the stuff your dentist scrapes off your teeth during your regular cleanings). What's the big deal with tartar? Nothing if you're talking about the sauce you serve with fish. But tartar on your teeth is a whole other story. Contrary to what some would have you believe, tartar is *not* a protective layer over your teeth.

Plaque begins to form right after it is removed—as in five minutes after it's removed! That's why frequent brushing is important to prevent tartar formation. Once tartar is formed, it's like the bad bacteria are now cemented on your teeth. Only a pro can take that literal shit off.

So, being that plaque is easily removed and tartar must be scraped off by a professional—you can probably tell where I'm going with this—we can (more like "ought to") brush off the plaque before it becomes damaging tartar and sidestep the entire issue.

BEYOND BRUSHING

Brush, floss, rinse! Just those three things alone, done properly twice every day, will greatly improve your oral health. But the point of this book is to help you get the *healthiest* mouth possible, because that is what will make your whole body healthier and your wallet lighter from savings on medical costs. To achieve that goal, we need to look beyond what we can do specific to the mouth and focus on the lifestyle changes we can make in general that will support our oral health.

CHAPTER 11

The Whole Body and Nothing but the Whole Body

PROBABLY ONE OF THE MOST EFFECTIVE WAYS TO IMPROVE your health is by eating well. I mean, yes, you should stop smoking and drinking, start sleeping well, and exercise, but if we give some priority to foods that promote good oral health, we'll set up the rest of our body to be even healthier!

Those foods include lots of vegetables and fresh fruit and some animal proteins. If that sounds similar to a paleo style of eating, that's because it is. And that is something I highly recommend. If that is too extreme for you, then the minimum you should aim for is avoiding processed foods and refined grains.

Vegetables are good for our oral health because they are high in fiber, which feeds the good bacteria in our bodies. Their fibrous nature also helps clean the plaque off our teeth. And they are full of vitamins and antioxidants, like vitamin C, which increase our immunity, reduce our chances of getting infections, and protect our tissues from oxidative stress.

Vegetables should make up 50 percent of our total diet. Want to burn some calories without going to the gym? It takes more calories to digest vegetables than are in them! And the fiber in those vegetables slows down sugar absorption, which is super important for blood glucose control.

Animal proteins are fine to eat as long as they are from good sources (organic, grass-fed, free-range, no hormones or antibiotics, you know the drill). I realize there are people who think eating meat is unhealthy because they have problems digesting meat products. Often that's related to them having insufficient enzymes, so they wind up with a more-or-less rotting cesspool of putrid animal products in their guts (gross!). If you have difficulty digesting animal products or feel unwell after eating them, you can supplement them with enzymes.

Protein is the most important thing in our diets because proteins are the building blocks for all of our cellular functions. In other words, do not be protein deficient if you want a healthy body. If you are plant-based, be sure to consume enough protein from seeds, nuts, beans, lentils, and supplements.

Those seeds, nuts, and beans will also help you get the healthy fats you need. Fat is a vital component for a healthy saliva pellicle; therefore, eating healthy fats like avocado is important.

Many people have issues with gluten and dairy. Those foods can destroy the GI tract and cause inflammation. If you are unsure if you can tolerate gluten and dairy, look for signs of inflammation. Is your poop healthy and regular? Do you have achy joints? Are your gums bleeding? If the answer to these questions is yes, try avoiding both and see if you notice improvements in those areas.

Regardless of what type of diet you do eat, you're probably not getting optimum levels of nutrients. It's an ironic fact of life in modern times: we have more food than ever on this planet, yet almost all of us are nutrient deficient in one way or another. Because of that, I often recommend supplements.

NEED A LITTLE SUPPLEMENTAL HELP?

I would have to write an encyclopedia if I were going to talk about every nutrient you need. Since this book is about your mouth, I'm just going to focus on what most of us need to support our oral health.

The first thing I want to talk about is pre- and probiotics.

The distinction between prebiotics and probiotics is that probiotics contain the actual good bacteria that you want inside of you—they are what build a strong and healthy microbiome (both the one in your gut and the one in your mouth). Prebiotics, on the other hand, feed the good bacteria that is already existing in your microbiome.

Lots of people are already aware of probiotics (who isn't eating yogurt for gut health these days?). But you need both.

The "big two" of the prebiotic world are inulin (dietary soluble fiber found in plants such as artichokes, onions, garlic, bananas, asparagus, and leeks and the supplement Benefiber) and xylitol (you'll soon learn about this natural sweetener, a.k.a., a busy miracle worker).

To give a little empirical evidence, there was a study conducted to assess the effect of pre- and probiotics on oral health. Results showed that probiotics can help neutralize acidic mouths, preventing the growth of cariogenic bacteria. The results also revealed that patients with gingivitis, periodontitis, and similar problems had improved their gum health after chewing prebiotic chewing gums (i.e., xylitol gum that neutralizes your mouth). And using probiotic-based mouthwashes also prevented the growth of sulfur-based bacteria, leading to odor-free breath.[75]

Look for oral probiotics containing these strains to maximize your oral health supplementation:

- *Lactobacillus reuteri*
- *Lactobacillus salivarius*
- *Streptococcus salivarius* K12
- *Streptococcus salivarius* M18
- *Lactobacillus paracasei*
- *Lactobacillus sakei*

All pre- and probiotics are excellent for your oral microbiome and your gut microbiome, which I've spoken about at length. You probably know by now that if you take care of them, they will take care of you. Taking care of them means being sure that in addition to the pre- and probiotics, you also abide by the well-balanced, whole-food diet I just spoke about, *and* you aren't so freaking clean that you're killing off all the good bacteria your probiotics are feeding.

WHAT MAKES A TOOTH

I feel a vital part of understanding the importance of pro-oral health supplements actually comes from understanding the structure of our teeth (it's more than a white chunky rock in your mouth). Understanding the tooth's build allows us to see

---

75   Jørn A. Aas et al., "Defining the Normal Bacterial Flora of the Oral Cavity," *Journal of Clinical Microbiology* 43, no. 11 (November 2005): 5721–5732, https://doi.org/10.1128/JCM.43.11.5721-5732.2005.

what exactly we are assisting in our efforts. We'll work from the outside in.

Up first is the enamel—this is the hard, white outer layer that we all see and know. The enamel is actually dead (which is why it can't repair itself) and is 97 percent hydroxyapatite (a composition of calcium and phosphate, as mentioned earlier). This is very much a protective layer and is the hardest substance in our bodies. That fact alone should open your eyes to the seriousness of breaking a tooth; if your enamel is harder than your femur, what the hell were you doing with your teeth if you broke one?

Under that layer is the dentin (get it? I'm a *den*-tist?), which can repair the enamel (the dentin is alive). However, the dentin can only repair the most minute of insults. Let me make that super clear. I am not saying you can reverse cavities or heal major problems on your own; once you have an actual hole in your tooth, it's irreversible, and you need professional help. A large portion of the dentin is made up of odontoblast cells, which serve to protect the pulp (the lifeline) of the tooth. When bacteria do make their way through the enamel, the odontoblast releases an immune response that kills the bacteria before the buggers reach the pulp. The other major portion of the dentin's makeup is the same hydroxyapatite material as in the enamel. But being that this is only around 70 percent of it, the dentin is much softer (and more vulnerable) than the enamel.

Lastly, and already mentioned, is the pulp—the heartbeat of the tooth. Here, you'll find the nerves and blood supply of the tooth. So, naturally, this is the area where you feel pain when there's a problem. This brings up a good point. Oftentimes when I tell my patients that I've found a problem, they'll respond with "But I don't feel it." That's good! That means the infection hasn't reached the pulp yet. Once bacteria reach the deepest layer of your tooth, my options as an oral healthcare provider become severely limited (root canals and extractions mainly). A root canal essentially kills the tooth, as the nerve and blood supply to it are removed. While many patients and clinicians have strong feelings about root canals, I am not here to dive into that debate. Rather, I'm simply saying that when the pulp is infected, it is one of the two options.

The definition of an organ is a group of tissues working together to perform a specific function. Thus our teeth are organs, and thus we must take care of them as if they were our heart/liver/pancreas/brain. If you were going to lose a liver, wouldn't you want to replace it?

When someone doesn't have an oral health–focused diet, it harms their enamel. When someone doesn't correct the problem with their enamel, bacteria get through the dentin, infect the pulp, and cause problems throughout the body. And when oral issues start popping up elsewhere in the body, Dr. Lee writes a book explaining why that's happening.

Our teeth are constantly doing battle: protecting the pulp and repairing themselves. This is why dead teeth (teeth with root canals or abscessed teeth) develop decay and periodontal disease faster than living teeth—they have nothing to repair themselves with.

The composition of teeth is important to know because we must also care for our teeth from the inside out with our diet and supplements, if necessary (and they usually are necessary).

OTHER PRO-TOOTH SUPPLEMENTS

One supplement that's critical for odontoblast function is

vitamin D_3, obtained from daily small exposures to the sun or through supplementation. An added benefit: it's antiviral!

Vitamin D_3 is actually a hormone, not a vitamin. Semantics! Nearly all, if not all, cells in the body have receptors for D_3, which is why this hormone/vitamin is so important. If you are experiencing a lot of cavities and your diet and oral care routines are in check, be sure to get your D_3 levels screened. You may be insufficient.

Increasing your D_3 intake is good anyway, as most people are deficient in it. Plus, it is also anti-inflammatory and anti-carcinogenic, helps with gut digestion and metabolism, and helps bring calcium to your bones and teeth, increasing their strength. However, the calcium must be directed; otherwise it takes the path of least resistance and gets dumped into your soft tissues such as arteries (causing hardened arteries, leading to heart disease), your kidneys (causing kidney stones), or your gallbladder (causing gallstones). Luckily, we have vitamin K_2, which can lead calcium to be placed where it ought to be, namely in our teeth and bones. (This explains why people with osteoporosis who just take calcium without K_2 wind up with hardened arteries.)

Because of its calcium deposition abilities, supplementation of K_2 alone creates a 60 percent reduction in vertebral fractures and an 80 percent reduction in hip and nonvertebral fractures.[76] D_3 and K_2 vitamins are available for purchase, or you can go straight to the source and get them by eating grass-fed animal food sources (grass has vitamin K_1 which, when digested by animals, is converted into K_2).

---

76 Trasey D. Falcone, Scott S. W. Kim, and Megan H. Cortazzo, "Vitamin K: Fracture Prevention and Beyond," *PM&R* 3, no. 6S (2011): S82–87, https://doi.org/10.1016/j.pmrj.2011.04.008.

Tartar isn't always a sign of poor oral hygiene. I've had several patients come in swearing they brush and floss every day (I often believe the brushing part), yet their teeth are covered in tartar. Usually, that means they have an excess of calcium in their saliva instead of in their bones, where it belongs. I often recommend those patients take some vitamin K_2, as that's what helps the calcium they're getting in their diet get into their bones.

Vitamin A is another great supplement that supports bone and teeth. It is involved in keratin formation. Keratin is found in enamel. Vitamin A works by inducing cell differentiation into osteoblasts and supports osteoclast formation (it helps build up the new bone and tear down the old). Retinol and beta-carotene are sources of vitamin A and are commonly found in orange foods like oranges and sweet potatoes.

Another important nutrient is vitamin C. Did you know that humans cannot make their own vitamin C? We must ensure we get enough of it from our diets or through supplementation so that we don't end up like those sailors whose teeth fell out. Vitamin C is important for tissue and collagen building, so it plays a leading role in preventing and managing periodontitis and in wound healing (this is especially important if you are going to have surgery). It is a powerful antioxidant, helps us with stress management, and is a natural antiviral and antibacterial.

My favorite supplement is magnesium. This mineral is crucial to our survival, and most people, if not all, are deficient. The reason we are deficient is because this mineral is destroyed by stress, and I know very few people who can say they are not stressed. (So if you are at a stressful time in your life, up your magnesium intake!) Magnesium activates our D_3 (which is important for heart health as it regulates our heartbeat), improves our insulin sensitivity, and helps us detox. However, the reason why magnesium is my favorite is that it helps us sleep and poop better! It also relaxes muscles, so I recommend it to all of my patients who grind their teeth. For best results, take it at night before bed.

Lastly, a few great anti-inflammatory supplements to consider include fish oil and algae oil, and curcumin. The omega-3 fatty acids found in fish and algae oil are vital for health and are not produced in our bodies. They lower heart disease and blood pressure, lower triglycerides and cholesterol, help prevent cognitive decline, help the immune system, aid digestion, and increase fertility. They are found in fish, flax seeds, chia seeds, or store-bought supplements. Curcumin is the bright yellow spice found in turmeric and is commonly used in Indian cuisine (think curry). This stuff is a *potent* anti-inflammatory but not easily absorbed, so combine it with black pepper for better absorption.

As for the proper amounts of these supplements, consult with your doctor. You can have your levels tested to get a baseline, but everyone is different and needs a different amount accordingly.

"So, Dr. Lee, if I take all these supplements, can I eat cake for breakfast?"

Um, no. Sugar is still sugar. It's the antithesis of everything related to good oral health. But I get it. I have a sweet tooth too. Thankfully, there are great sugar substitutes.

Ever wonder why you crave sugar? It's because when you eat sugar and processed foods, it feeds the bad bacteria in your gut microbiome and encourages their growth. And as those sugar-loving bacteria grow, they require more and more sugar to support themselves, hence the cravings.

FAUX SUGAR

You know sugar's bad for you in general. And you know it's bad for your teeth. It's nothing but a cavity-causing bunch of empty calories. The cavities come because bacteria *thrive* on sugar—the fastest way to build a bad biofilm is by putting sugar in your mouth.

But a good dessert is like that bad boy or girl you had a crush on in high school. No matter what your mother said, you just couldn't stay away. What's a good flosser to do?

Dabble with xylitol.

Xylitol is a good sugar substitute that has a superpower: it will actually combat bacteria like *Strep. mutans*, which metabolize xylitol.[77] They eat it and yet starve to death.

Meanwhile, *Strep. mutans* can still metabolize other sugar as well as sugar substitutes and artificial sweeteners like Sweet'N Low, Splenda, and stevia (granted, not as much as it can Imperial cane sugar). So if you love your sweets, look for those with xylitol as a sugar substitute.

So now you know: a good diet that supports your oral health is one where you lean toward plant-based foods, supplement appropriately, and limit sugar. If you want to really take your diet to level eleven, you go one step further and try intermittent fasting.

FASTING

Here's proof I'm human: I'm a habitual snacker. I love to graze all the days. Used to, actually. I don't anymore because I kept getting cavities (yes, dentists get cavities too!)

---

77   Yukako Kojima et al., "Combining Prebiotics and Probiotics to Develop Novel Synbiotics that Suppress Oral Pathogens," *Journal of Oral Biosciences* 58, no. 1 (February 2016): 27–32, https://doi.org/10.1016/j.job.2015.08.004.

If you're a grazer, you might have something similar going on in your mouth, even if you're grazing on fruit and nuts, things that aren't normally associated with cavities. That's because grazing makes it hard for your mouth to maintain a healthy pH. We'll cover more on pH in a minute; for now, it's important to remember that your mouth's pH level decreases when you eat.

After eating, your mouth's pH drops to around 5.5. This is true for any food, even things like celery and carrots because it helps our body digest the food. (Though if you must snack, raw veggies are the recommended choice. Their crunchiness helps clean your teeth.) It takes about an hour for the pH to return to normal, and then your saliva will start putting minerals back in your teeth.

If you are consistently eating throughout the day, your mouth is always acidic and constantly demineralizing. For this reason (and a host of other good ones), fasting between meals is extremely beneficial; long lengths of time between eating puts your mouth in an alkaline state where your saliva rebuilding your teeth is a godsend.

Fasting is important for blood glucose levels too. When we eat, sugar goes into our blood, and insulin needs time to take that glucose into our cells. If we are constantly eating, there is a constant supply of new sugar floating around our body waiting for insulin to store away the earlier influx of it. As that analogy from Chapter 4 points out, sugar in our blood acts like shards of glass in our vessels, which causes our vessels to become inflamed. Right, snacking can lead to inflammation. Fasting doesn't.

ABOUT THAT PH THING

I've mentioned oral pH a few times now, and feel I owe a better explanation of how it works and why it's important. Essentially, our mouths like to stay at a neutral pH between 6.2 and 7.2, which is perfect because we want our mouths—and bodies—to be as neutral as possible or even slightly alkaline. Why? Because disease thrives in an acidic environment.

The pH in our mouths changes as we eat because many of the foods and liquids we consume are acidic (just think of the citric acid in fruit or the tangy flavor of tomatoes, and don't get me started on sodas). These obviously change the mouth to be more acidic. However, even food that is basic (a pH greater than 7) will increase the mouth's acidity as well at first. While eating, our saliva releases enzymes (amylase) that start to break down our food (the first stage of digestion). As part of that process, these enzymes drop the pH of our mouths, beginning about fifteen minutes after we start eating.

If you must drink something acidic, it is best to drink it all at once and through a straw. Be sure to rinse your mouth out with water afterward to eliminate as much of the acid as possible. The worst thing you can do is sip on a soda all day long.

This process also weakens the enamel on your teeth (later remineralized by saliva). Because of this, you should wait thirty to sixty minutes after eating before brushing your teeth. The same goes for after throwing up! (Looking at you, pregnant moms.)

Something I recommend to my patients is xylitol chewing gum. Not only does it kill the *Strep. mutans* bacteria, but it also stimulates saliva, thereby increasing the mouth's pH and preventing demineralization (and it strengthens the masticatory muscles—your chewing ones—which support bone health).

Interestingly, everything I've spoken about in this section on what makes a good oral health diet—plant-based menu, supplements, abstaining from sugar, and intermittent fasting—all have something else in common. They are anti-inflammatory. See how it all comes full circle? What's good for the goose's mouth is also good for the goose's body.

Other anti-inflammatory lifestyle practices are also likewise good for your oral health. Let's look at a few of them now.

OPEN UP AND SAY OM

Stress impacts every aspect of your health because it is inflammatory, so one way to stay healthy is just to never get stressed—which, yeah, I know is impossible. What's not impossible is to counter all the stressful events and activities in your life with things that relieve stress. Yoga and meditation or breathing exercises are the first practices I often recommend.

There is so much science out there about how yoga and meditation reduce stress and anxiety.[78] Once part of a regular practice, many people find it improves their mood and sense of well-being. Additionally, it helps your body grow stronger and more flexible. So why not do yoga or meditate? We all can sit and do nothing for ten minutes. Tell your spouse it's doctor's orders.

A key part of yoga is being aware of your breath as you move

---

78 Kristen E. Riley and Crystal L. Park, "How Does Yoga Reduce Stress? A Systematic Review of Mechanisms of Change and Guide to Future Inquiry," *Health Psychology Review* 9, no. 3 (2015): 379–396, https://doi.org/10.1080/17437199.2014.981778; Mahesh Narain Tripathi, Sony Kumari, and Tikhe Sham Ganpat, "Psychophysiological Effects of Yoga on Stress in College Students," *Journal of Education and Health Promotion* 7, no. 43 (2018): 43, https://www.jehp.net/article.asp?issn=2277-9531;year=2018;volume=7;issue=1;spage=43;epage=43;aulast=Tripathi;type=0.

into, move out of, and hold positions while breathing through your nose. Nose breathing has an amazing benefit! Our noses release nitric oxide (NO) as we inhale, which then enters our airways and lungs. NO is a vasodilator, meaning it dilates our blood vessels. That's a good thing. Constricted blood vessels often go hand in hand with high blood pressure, which is probably one of the reasons why mouth breathers typically have high blood pressure. Even if you don't have hypertension, the NO is helpful because that nasal air has about a 10 to 15 percent higher oxygen content than mouth-breathed air.

Aim for at least five minutes of stress-relieving breathing every day. Take long, slow, and deep breaths—breathing into your belly—through your nose for five minutes. I don't care how busy you are; you can find five minutes to do this. Try it first thing in the morning or right before bed.

There are some amazing apps you can download on your phone that will walk you through many different types of breathing. Just search for "breathwork" or "meditation" on your phone's app store.

A few of my favorite apps are Breathe, Calm, Headspace, and Othership.

My favorite stress-relieving breathing technique is called boxed breathing: inhale for a count of four, hold for four, exhale for four, hold for four, repeat.

Alleviating stress will also help with your sleep architecture, meaning you'll get better sleep. And good sleep architecture is another anti-inflammatory strategy.

SLEEP LIKE A VAMPIRE

I don't have to tell you this; you know it already. But because you're probably not doing it, I'm going to say it anyway:

Get eight hours of sleep every night.

Eight hours is just one-third of your day. Think about it: vampires can come out after sundown. Meanwhile, they sleep all day, which means they're averaging twelve hours! And look at their teeth! Beautiful white fangs. Proof sleep equals good teeth.

Okay, yes, I'm getting carried away. But I have your attention now. So I'll get on with it.

Sleep does more than just clear up under-eye bags. The cells in our brains temporarily shrink when we get into a deep enough sleep, which is what allows the glymphatic system to wash away any buildup of neurotoxins and beta-amyloid plaques (those things that, when left to build up in our brains, are considered a hallmark of Alzheimer's). Sleep is also crucial for helping us solidify the things we learned during the day and store the new memories in a place where we can find them later.

All that, and it helps with oral health too, which is pretty amazing.

One way sleep helps you have a healthier mouth is because sleep deprivation is associated with inflammation. When you don't get enough sleep, your body responds by increasing inflammatory molecules, including cytokines, C-reactive protein (something that, when elevated, flags people at risk for heart disease and diabetes), and our old nemesis, interleukin 6.[79]

The other way good sleep benefits oral health is by helping to keep your cortisol levels within normal limits. When we stress our bodies by not getting enough sleep, our adrenals pump out cortisol to give us energy. But cortisol doesn't create energy

---

79 "How Sleep Deprivation Can Cause Inflammation," Harvard Health Publishing, Harvard Medical School, January 11, 2022, https://www.health.harvard.edu/sleep/how-sleep-deprivation-can-cause-inflammation.

by pulling it out of a top hat; it needs a fuel of some kind. The fastest fuel to convert to energy is sugar, which explains why we tend to crave carbohydrates (sugar) when we're tired; from sugar, our bodies get the energy they need to read emails in the middle of the afternoon.

By this point, I don't think I have to explain why refined carbs or sugar are bad for your teeth. So get some sleep!

Easier said than done, I know. If you're having difficulty, see your dentist or regular physical doctor to get a sleep study done to rule out OSA. Up to 67 percent percent of insomnia patients have OSA, and they just don't know it.[80] Yet, if left untreated, OSA can become the most damaging condition for your health. It can lead to dementia—just one night of bad sleep can cause beta-amyloid plaques to form in the brain! And untreated OSA can take ten to fifteen years off your life. That's worse than what diabetes and smoking will do to you.[81]

While I'm urging you to go see a doctor if you're having trouble sleeping, try not to accept a pill for an answer. Many people tell their PCPs they're having trouble sleeping or that they think they have anxiety and depression, and their docs write a prescription for Ambien to help them sleep and trazodone to deal with the anxiety or depression (which is often a direct result of insomnia). Yes, those drugs do some good for some people, but you really should get to the root of why you're not sleeping.

Sure, on the surface, a sedative seems like it would kill two birds with one stone: you'll sleep, which will help resolve the anxiety and depression. You must get tested for OSA before you

80   Faith S. Luyster, Daniel J. Buysse, and Patrick J. Strollo, Jr., "Comorbid Insomnia and Obstructive Sleep Apnea: Challenges for Clinical Practice and Research," *Journal of Clinical Sleep Medicine* 6, no. 2 (2010): 196–204, https://pubmed.ncbi.nlm.nih.gov/20411700/.

81   Johns Hopkins Medicine, "Obstructive Sleep Apnea," accessed April 25, 2023, https://www.hopkinsmedicine.org/health/conditions-and-diseases/obstructive-sleep-apnea.

agree to any kind of sedative. Should you stop breathing in your sleep due to OSA, your body will do whatever it can to wake you up so that you do breathe again. Sedatives can override that arousal system.[82] Do you know what's worse than sleeping through your alarm clock on the day you have a massive presentation at work? Sleeping through your body's attempt to wake you up and tell you you're not breathing. That will get you to your funeral a little earlier than you'd ever planned.

Wondering if you might have OSA? Here are some frequent symptoms:

- Drowsiness/low energy
- Anxiety/depression/mood instability
- High blood pressure
- Erectile dysfunction
- ADHD
- Sugar and/or caffeine cravings
- Bad breath
- Scalloped tongue
- Snoring
- Night terrors
- Frequent awakening and/or urination at night
- GERD
- Morning headaches when you're not hungover
- Migraines
- Bruxism (teeth grinding)
- Tornado bed—you know, when you wake up and it looks like a tornado happened in your bed

---

82 Barry Krakow, Victor A. Ulibarri, and Natalia D. McIver, "Pharmacotherapeutic Failure in a Large Cohort of Patients with Insomnia Presenting to a Sleep Medicine Center and Laboratory: Subjective Pretest Predictions and Objective Diagnoses," *Mayo Clinic Proceedings* 89, no. 12 (December 2014): 1608–1620, https://doi.org/10.1016/j.mayocp.2014.04.032.

If you have a night guard, you should consider doing a sleep test because if the grinding is caused by sleep apnea, then wearing a night guard will make the apnea worse because it reduces the tongue space even more.

While everyone with chronic insomnia should get checked by a doctor, occasional sleepless nights happen to us all and are not a concern as long as the "occasional" adjective stays true. When that happens, if you're in a pinch, try an all-natural supplement like melatonin or magnesium or run a warm bath with lavender oil in it to help you settle down or meditate.

Meanwhile, develop good sleep hygiene habits. That means:

- Create a boring sleep ritual that includes going to bed and getting up around the same time every day.
- No glowing screens (phones, tablets, e-readers, TVs, computers, etc.) for an hour before you go to bed.
- Keep your room dark—no lights.
- Keep your room on the cool side; between sixty-two and sixty-seven degrees is ideal for sleeping.
- Cut the caffeine out of your day at 3:00 p.m., and eliminate alcohol for at least three hours and food for two hours before going to bed.

Your sleep habits, like your food choices and how you manage your oral care are all under your control. That means taking steps to improve and secure your oral health is all up to you. Each step you take and follow through on for your Personal Wellness Plan is totally your choice—your choice for better health, for keeping more money in your pocket, and for a longer life.

But you'll still need to do that thing at least twice a year (preferably four times): go see your dentist.

MAINTAIN YOUR BRAIN

In Chapter 9, I promised solutions to help protect your brain to prevent dementia. To that end, the following is a list of brain-healthy activities. Some, you'll notice, are what you need to do for your overall health in general. Others you may be delighted to find that you *want* to incorporate into your life. I mean, who doesn't want to eat a little chocolate on doctor's (dentist's!) orders?

So here are my top tips to maintain a healthy brain and stave off Alzheimer's and dementia:

1. Avoid sugar and processed foods; keep your blood glucose levels under control.
2. Eat fish to get your omega-3 fatty acids, or supplement with fish or algae oil.
3. Indulge in dark chocolate! At 70 percent cocoa, dark chocolate is rich in flavanols and antioxidants. It's actually good for your heart and your brain.
4. Get regular exercise; movement increases blood flow to the brain.
5. Be social: hanging out with others and companionship stimulates our brains.
6. Work on improving your sleep hygiene, and get the amount of sleep you need (seven to eight hours every night).
7. Supplement your diet, in addition to the omega-3 already mentioned, with choline, a vitamin B complex, vitamin D, and zinc.
8. Mind your gut! Your gut is responsible for 95 percent of the production of neurotransmitters that are used in the brain.

9. Keep your stress in check—engage in mediation.
10. Challenge your thinking. Keep your brain active through puzzles and games that require strategy, reading, and good conversations.

A LITTLE MORE THAN JUST BRUSHING
GET TO KNOW YOUR DENTIST

You know how your insurance pays for two teeth cleanings a year? That's not enough. Really, seeing your dentist four times a year is the best practice. Before you balk at that, think it through: it's just four hours out of a year. You spend more than that shopping each week. (In case you're interested, the average person spends ten hours a week shopping![83])

Those four hours in the chair are when your dentist can talk to you about how to improve your systemic health. That's when they will find evidence to make an early diagnosis of chronic disease before it causes irreversible harm. And that's when they will discover and treat your gingivitis.

It's important to tackle gingivitis as early as possible because, in those first stages of the disease, it is curable! Otherwise, you can risk developing periodontitis, which puts you at a 23 to 46 percent higher chance of dying from heart issues than people who don't have the disease.[84]

In fact, your dentist can catch *all* oral diseases early! Since they are much cheaper to treat than a related catastrophe six months (or longer) down the road, why not suck it up and just

---

83   Dan Kopf, "Americans Spend Two Hours Less a Month on Shopping than They Did 15 Years Ago," Quartz, July 31, 2019, https://qz.com/1677747/americans-are-spending-way-less-time-shopping/.

84   Vivenca Wallin Bengtsson et al., "Periodontitis Related to Cardiovascular Events and Mortality: A Long-Time Longitudinal Study," *Clinical Oral Investigations* 25 (2021): 4085–4095, https://doi.org/10.1007/s00784-020-03739-x.

go to the dentist more often? After all, gingivitis can set in in as little as five days! If you develop it and wait six months to have it taken care of at your next cleaning (and you are like the majority of the population and don't floss daily or brush like you should, eat poorly, and are stressed), you will wind up spending much much more. A typical gingivitis cleaning is around $150, whereas a periodontal disease cleaning is around $1,000. So if you want to save money, go to the dentist sooner and more frequently.

I can hear you now: "But my insurance doesn't pay for cleanings four times a year."

Well, honey, insurance is not there for your benefit. They are a for-profit business.

And if saving money isn't enough of an incentive, a 2021 study from the *Journal of Clinical Periodontology* reported that patients with gum disease were nine times (NINE TIMES) more likely to die from COVID-19. They were also three times more likely to be admitted to a hospital and four and a half times more likely to require the assistance of a ventilator. Why the increased risk? Because of the inflammation caused by periodontal disease.[85]

IS YOUR DENTIST DR. RIGHT?

You have to be able to trust your doctor. That trust is, in part, built on being able to establish a good rapport with them, which often begins with them expressing an interest in your overall health and well-being. Here's what to look for to be certain you have the right dentist for you.

---

85   "Gum Disease Linked to COVID-19 Complications," *BDJ Team* 8, no. 5 (2021), https://doi.org/10.1038/ s41407-021-0604-1.

- Are they taking a very detailed medical history of you and your family?
- Are they asking about your lifestyle and diet choices?
- Are they measuring your gums *every time* you go in?
- Are they educating you on things you can do in your life to be healthier?
- Are you experiencing dental emergencies between visits, like breaking teeth or getting toothaches or bleeding gums?
- Do you feel better and healthier in general after visiting your dentist?
- Are they just telling you to brush and floss better without providing treatment options to stop the bleeding gums?

And on top of that, there's all the stuff I mentioned earlier that your dentist could be doing: DNA tests on your saliva for bacteria strains, CBCT scans, any of the genetic tests that could shed light on what's happening in your body, or even the VELscope.

The point is, your dentist is there for more than just making sure you have a pretty smile. You should take advantage of everything they can offer you. Your whole body will benefit from it!

In between your regular visits to the dentist, though, there are a few things to be aware of in your mouth that should inspire you to make an impromptu appointment.

- If you have a nonhealing lesion in your mouth—one that lasts for more than two weeks—you should get it checked out.
- If you feel lumps or bumps in new places that, again, last longer than two weeks, have your dentist take a look-see.

Even if the lumps are painless, get them looked at; it's often the things that don't hurt that are cancerous.

- If you're experiencing signs you may be grinding your teeth at night, maybe new jaw pain, your teeth feel worn, or you're waking up in the middle of the night or waking up in the morning with a headache, go speak to someone about the possibility of sleep apnea.
- If your gums start to bleed when brushing or flossing
- If there is a foul odor in your mouth

As you can see, good oral health is more than a matter of proper brushing and flossing. Truly, it's an entire lifestyle change that's needed. But you're not in this alone! You have a dentist nearby who's eager to help you on your journey to the healthiest life you can imagine. Let's look at what the oral care community can do for you, beginning with testing.

CHAPTER 12

Let's Get Testing

IN THIS CHAPTER, I WANT TO GO OVER OTHER FORMS OF testing that your dentist can do to see what's going on in your mouth that is causing, or may eventually cause, disease.

Diagnostic testing is important to obtain objective results. Formerly, dentistry was largely a subjective field, basing diagnoses of decay and disease on what was seen, not measured. This approach created ambiguity between patients and dentists and caused confusion when professionals disagreed on a diagnosis. Quantified testing has revolutionized the oral health world, giving a solid baseline from which to track progress over time. You would do well to see a dentist that adheres to this objective philosophy.

More and more objective testing and diagnostics are coming to the market every day. Soon, AI will be the norm in helping dentists diagnose conditions off of radiographs and imaging.

THE TESTS THEMSELVES

Off the bat, we have a number of relatively simple tests (all done in a dentist's office) that are extremely helpful, such as:

- Oral Microbiome testing (e.g., OralDNA® Alert 2™): a genetic IL-6 (interleukin) and oral bacteria test
  - If you're unlucky in the genes department, you might be like me and have the IL-6 mutation marker. That tells you you're more prone to having an inflammatory response than most other people. Our bodies release interleukin proteins to help regulate cell growth, differentiation, and mobility. Interleukins also play an important role in necessary inflammation—as in the kind to ward off infection. However, if you are born (like I was) with an IL-6 gene mutation, your body is preset to be in an inflammatory state—with a relatively small insult, you will have an abnormally intense immune response and higher levels of inflammation. Because we all want to keep inflammation to a minimum, knowing you have this marker will enable you and your dentist to be proactive and try to prevent inflammation before it starts.
  - The bacterial microbiome test will find and name all the "wonderful" bad actor bacteria present in your mouth, as well as how they are affecting other organ systems. Knowing what's there will help your dentist tailor the appropriate treatment to kill the bacteria.
- MMP-8 test: a diagnostic test for MMP-8 enzyme levels (responsible for breaking down connective tissues in the body). High levels of this enzyme mean you're having an inflammatory response and degradation going on. Sometimes we don't see that happening with our naked eyes until it's a full-blown in-your-face nasty infection. This test, how-

ever, is eighteen months predictive of a future breakdown in the mouth and allows the dentist to know the process is occurring before it appears on a radiograph or is seen clinically. It's all about proactive versus reactive care here, and discovering the degradation at an earlier time will help us treat it before things really deteriorate. The MMP-8 test is hard to find and not available everywhere in the US...yet, but it is used in Europe.

- HbA1c test: a blood sugar test (not all states allow dentists to test A1C, but all can test for blood sugar levels)
- *Strep. mutans* bacterial test: a simple test that looks for the bacteria that cause cavities, helping determine cavity risk
- HPV salivary test: saliva can be tested for HPV, which is important for oral cancer detection.
- Chairside bacterial tests: dentists can use a microscope to examine the types of bacteria in a patient's mouth chairside. This will let the dentist know if you have the type of bacteria responsible for gum disease.

There's a myth that some people are just genetically more prone to develop cavities. Don't get me wrong; there are a few genetic disorders that weaken the enamel (such as amelogenesis imperfecta), but those are exceedingly rare. If someone is doing what they need to at home for their oral health, they shouldn't get more cavities. At most, families "pass down" the same bad oral bacteria by sharing life together.

Those tests look for things found in samples of your saliva or blood. Outside of them, we have tests requiring tools that give us a better view of you physically.

THE VELSCOPE: ORAL ABNORMALITY SCREENING DEVICE

Ah, my old friend the VELscope. This tool is absolutely amazing. Like in the stories I've told, it's helped me help lots of people. While it doesn't detect cancer or other diseases per se, it does reveal what's going on subsurface and allows more diagnostics from there. The mouth's anatomy is just so strange (and colored red) already that a big flashlight that can highlight problem areas is worth its weight in gold. Oral cancer, in particular, tends to start in the throat or floor of the mouth, hidden from sight. By the time your dentist can see an issue with their overhead light, it's too late; you're already in stage 3 or 4 (the main reason that oral cancer survival rates have remained low, around 60 percent, and even if you do survive, you're living with part of your face missing. Who wants to do that?).

Now, there are other tools that do the same thing (I just love this one, plus it's radiation free!). The point is to make sure your dentist is using something other than the overhead light to check for cancer.

CBCT: 3D IMAGING

For years, dentists were limited to two-dimensional X-rays of teeth. X-rays were done at different angles to help try and build a better picture, but in the end, *teeth are still three-dimensional objects*. Enter cone-beam computed technology (CBCT), an advanced 3D imaging technique similar to a CT scan. This awesome technology allows clinicians to see 360 degrees around the tooth, thereby catching disease sooner. In addition, this scan doesn't use a wide range of radiation, as a CT scan does. It only uses a narrow cone (hence the name) on specified areas—all in all, a minor amount of radiation. Which, in reality, is completely negligible in comparison to seeing 30 to 40 percent more of the tooth. This allows dentists to catch asymptomatic chronic infections hiding in the bones or sinuses and treat them efficiently. It also allows the dentist to measure the volume of a patient's airway, which can help screen for sleep apnea and other airway health issues. Pretty cool, huh?!

If you're an X-ray-phobe, don't ignore this advice! Let me educate you on digital dental X-rays. These have 80 to 90 percent less radiation than traditional films and can help catch infections or diseases at the earliest stages, which is important for your health. Skipping X-rays, and therefore an early diagnosis, is more damaging for your health than receiving the X-rays. Dentists do not have X-ray vision, so asking them to do an exam without an X-ray to see beneath the surface is like asking a gastroenterologist to diagnose colon cancer without a colonoscopy. You can't diagnose what you can't see. If you want to cut back on your exposure to radiation, do so with things that can't save your health: reduce your time in airplanes, stop keeping your cell phone in your pocket, distance yourself from computer and TV screens, and don't use cat litter.

DIAGNOdent®

How does a radiation-free cavity detector sound? Pretty awesome, I know. And we have a tool that fits the bill: the DIAGNOdent. It's been around for a little while, but its accuracy in the past was not as good as I would want. However, it has improved dramatically.

It looks like a little pen, the end of which is put on a tooth to give you a reading. It won't tell you how deep a cavity has penetrated or how close to a nerve it is, nothing diagnostic like that. But it will say *yes* or *no* with zero radiation. Then if you get a *yes*, you can go on to other diagnostics to see if you have an abscess or whether a root canal is needed. In the future, AI will help us diagnose cavities with extreme precision. And I, for one, welcome our new robot overlords.

SLEEP TEST

I won't spend too much time here, as I wrote a whole chapter on it. Nevertheless, sleep tests are extremely useful in dentistry, and your dentist should be utilizing them or at least referring you to get one. For example, I had a patient in her early thirties who came in with bleeding gums. There wasn't much tartar on her teeth, and her saliva tests were negative for bacteria, so I knew the issue wasn't gum disease (not yet, at least) and suspected the issue was a result of mouth breathing. Her blood work came back fine as well. However, I noticed she was a teeth grinder and had TMJ headaches, so I had her complete an at-home sleep apnea test. Her apnea score came in below the diagnosis threshold (unobstructed snoring at worst), but her heart rate was spiking to over 140 beats per minute! Obviously, your heart rate should only spike this high during a workout. Her doctors were concerned about her being at risk for A-fib, and she was quickly placed on an arrhythmia medication by her primary doctor to balance out her heart rate. Long story short, her doctor sent me a thank-you note for finding the issue because they would have never known. (See? Just like the mouth to the body, I'm connecting the medical community as well!)

Dentists are always looking in the mouth, so it makes sense that they look at the airway and screen for signs of sleep apnea as well (most signs of apnea are associated with the mouth). The Mallampati score is a quick reference guide used to see that level, from Class I–Class IV, of sleep apnea risk someone has. It's an assessment that relates the size of the tongue to the opening of the throat. The classification is related to the risk of having sleep apnea.

In class I, you can see the entire airway, while in type IV, you cannot see any of the airway, as it is obstructed by the tongue. Patients who have class III and IV are at higher risk of having airway health issues.

Beyond this, simple tests of noticing inflamed tissue around the anterior teeth (mouth breathing), TMJ muscle hypertrophy (big chewing muscles from teeth grinding), and acid erosion (acid reflux) are enough to order an at-home sleep test. (Note: sleep apnea must be diagnosed by a physician.)

KEEP IT UP

Testing uncovers problems in their very early stages—that is, when they are easier to address. The other point is that once you're tested, you need to realize that your body changes, and you'll need to be tested again at regular intervals. The goal is always to catch things early. We have some amazing technology available to aid you in your health. Do yourself and your loved ones a favor and use it.

Or, if necessary, ask for it to be used on you. I want to take a moment and just say that if your dentist doesn't do everything I'm talking about, that doesn't mean they are a bad dentist! Some of the technologies that I've discussed are just coming into the world. If your dentist hasn't spoken to you about them yet, then maybe that means you should introduce them to these concepts and let them know you, as a patient, are very interested.

Now that you're familiar with the testing available, let's look at what else your dentist should be doing.

CHAPTER 13

Why Your Dentist
Is a Busybody

SOMETIMES, WHEN IT FEELS LIKE YOUR DENTIST HAS
three instruments and eight fingers in your mouth, they'll ask
you what you did on vacation. You should answer. We're trained
to understand what sounds like unintelligible conversation.
Besides, they do really want to know you as a human, not just
an open orifice full of teeth.

In fact, they should want to know all about you—possibly
in ways that make you think they're overstepping the boundary
separating them from other doctors. Trust me: they're not. A
good dentist should be a bit nosy when it comes to your whole
body's health and well-being. They should be doing things
that you might expect from your annual visits to your primary
care doctor (you do go to your primary care doctor every year,
right?).

~Insert sigh here.~

Your dentist should get a baseline on your health by checking your blood pressure and blood sugar, pry into your medical

history to learn about any habitual behaviors like smoking or a poor diet that could impact your health, and get a family medical history too. Family history, in particular, is *uber* important. Most of my patients are younger and don't yet have medical conditions or diagnoses. This could be because they are young, yes, or it could be because they just haven't gone to a doctor and had a diagnosis. After all, there are millions of diabetics walking around who have no idea their blood is sugar-saturated. A family history is vital because it tells us what you are at risk of developing.

Let's start at the beginning.

GET STRAPPED (INTO A CUFF)

Before anything happens in a dental office, someone should take your blood pressure. Someone meaning a hygienist or another member of the dental team, not some clown down the hall who's just being weird.

Few things piss me off more than hearing someone had a dental procedure without getting their blood pressure checked. Yet I hear about it so much, and it's become such a potential stressor that I'm frequently checking *my* blood pressure (thankfully, with yoga and breath exercises, my BP is pretty damn good).

If you're a healthy person, please don't think it's not a big deal if your dentist isn't doing this. It *is* a big deal—especially if you're a healthy person. Most people have no symptoms of an underlying health condition until the disease is in its later stages, which is when the damage has already occurred. So if you're the kind of person who sees their regular doctor once a year for an annual checkup (or every two or three years) because you're healthy and feel fine, you could be absolutely clueless about something brewing beneath the surface. Having your blood pressure checked every six months could be a quick and painless way of screening your health.

That's not even the primary reason your dentist should be checking your BP. If you're having some kind of work done that requires receiving an anesthetic, they should be strapping your arm in a pressure cuff and pumping it full of air so they don't cause you unnecessary trouble.

It's estimated that about one in three people who have high blood pressure don't know they do.[86] It's important to know if you do because anesthetics have epinephrine in them, which is essentially adrenaline. Adrenaline and high blood pressure don't make love connections. If a patient has high blood pressure— say they're regularly 150 over 100 or something like that—and their dentist gives them an injection with epinephrine, that could cause their blood pressure to spike and potentially give the patient a heart attack. Also, while the anesthetic is meant to go into the tissues surrounding the area where you are getting work done (it's not supposed to go into your bloodstream), we are injecting blindly and sometimes pierce a blood vessel. Even a small bit of epinephrine in the blood will cause a spike.

Aside from that potentially deadly event, high blood pressure can make patients bleed a lot during surgeries. So if a dentist knows that a person has high blood pressure prior to the surgery, they can be better prepared to handle the excess blood. Leaving a dentist's office on a stretcher is never a good look for anybody.

---

86   Salim S. Virani et al., "Heart Disease and Stroke Statistics—2020 Update: A Report from the American Heart Association," *Circulation* 141, no. 9 (2020): e139–e596, https://doi.org/10.1161/CIR.0000000000000757.

GIVE US SOME BLOOD (TESTING YOUR A1C)

Again, getting an A1C blood sugar check in the dentist's office isn't something that can happen in every state. However, more and more states are coming on board with the idea because it's benefiting patients for a few notable reasons. While dentists may not be able to check for A1C, they certainly can check with a meter that will tell you your current blood glucose level. One, it highlights patients who have undiagnosed glucose control problems, and two, it helps dentists better their care. For example, if a patient has undetected diabetes, that may explain why they have periodontal disease or gum issues and nonstop cavities—in fact, some people are discovering they might be diabetic *because* of that particular check by their dentist! If this information is known, we can then alter our treatment plans for these patients. I mean, it'd be good to know if the patient is diabetic so I can measure their glucose level prior to surgery and determine if they can heal afterward or not. That and, you know, make sure they don't wind up in a *diabetic coma...*

Whether it's just fainting in the dental chair (more common than you think from low blood sugar) or me deciding if I should perform surgery, knowing a patient's A1C levels helps me make better decisions regarding their care.

GETTING TO KNOW YOU

You wouldn't be the first patient to balk at the idea of having your BP taken or tested for your A1C/glucose level. I get it all the time from new patients. *Why are you doing this? I just need to get my teeth cleaned.* Or when I ask about how well they're sleeping, they'll push back, wanting to know why the hell it is any of my business because I'm just a dentist and not a "real" doctor.

At this point in the book, you know the answers. Because my patients haven't read it (at the time of this writing, anyway), I'll often preface my questions with a brief explanation about the mouth-body connection, which usually puts them at ease, and they'll be more likely to answer. And I usually begin by digging into their family's past.

LET'S TALK ABOUT YOUR MOTHER

It's important that your dentist knows about your family history. Often, they do this on the intake forms with a new patient; they have you check whether you or anyone in your family has a history of things like high blood pressure, high cholesterol, and so on.

Since no one's life ever remains static, your dentist or a member of their team should be checking in on that history during your exams to see if anything has changed since they last saw you. Maybe your mom didn't have high blood pressure until after teaching your kid sister how to drive, and now she's on medication for it. Your dentist needs to know. Whether it's a heart condition, a form of cancer, some systemic inflammation, or something else, that information needs to be passed on to your dentist. Yes, genes only count for a small percentage of disease manifestation, but they can provide clues to guide your dentist on what risk factors to look for and how things might progress over time.

Discussing your family history with you will help your dentist be proactive with your oral (whole body) health rather than relying on the X-rays you hate having done every year. Thinking about that is another thing that raises my hackles (and yet one more reason I practice what I preach and do breathwork!). Although necessary, X-rays encourage dentists to be reactive!

They provide two-dimensional photographs that tell us damage has already been done. I know we (the dentists) are doing the best we can with what we have, but traditionally, dentistry has been a reactive profession—only fixing problems once we can see them.

When your dentist is looking at your X-rays, they are looking at the densification or calcification of material in your teeth and bones. Meanwhile, it takes anywhere from six weeks to six months to see a change in density—that means six weeks to six months for a disease to be lurking before it's identified. So if you develop a cavity in your tooth shortly after having your annual X-rays completed, your dentist might not be able to see it for another year or even a little longer (because it was hard to squeeze that one-hour appointment into your calendar, I know!).

What many people don't realize is that dentistry is a pretty subjective profession. Dentists see something on an X-ray or in a patient's mouth, and we have to make an assumption or diagnosis based on what we see. There are few objective findings or test results to help us (which is one of the reasons why the saliva swabs are so exciting!). So we recommend treatment plans based on our experience.

Knowing a patient has a family history of diabetes, heart disease, dementia, or something else will give us a different lens to look through when we make our assumptions. If your dentist sees signs that destruction is occurring, and traditional X-rays aren't saying there's a problem, but you have a family history of a particular disease, then your doctor doesn't have to wait for the X-rays to confirm at a later date before formulating a customized treatment plan to hopefully prevent that disease.

Dental insurance poses another issue. While helpful in increasing access and affordability to care, it doesn't pay for all of the necessary tests and procedures needed to be proactive in your health journey. Just because it is not covered by insurance, does not mean that it is not needed!

NOW THAT YOU'RE IN THE CHAIR

Once your BP is taken and your dentist is caught up on the family dramas, it's time to get to the point of your visit: the actual exam. They'll probe around your mouth, measure your gums, examine your airway, do some tests, and hopefully send you on your way with a clean bill of health.

TIME FOR A LITTLE GUM PROBING

You should get your gums measured every time you visit your dentist. This is the poking exercise so many stupid memes are based on. (Yes, I've seen them.) We're not stabbing your gums to make them bleed. We're measuring the space, or pocket, between your gums and where they attach to your teeth. That pocket is an indicator of the health of your gums—the smaller it is, the healthier your gums.

People hate getting their gums measured. I know. Again, I've seen the memes. But even if your mouth looks beautiful to the naked eye and you're not suffering any symptoms, we have to do the measuring each time you visit us. First, that's because your oral health status can change in as little as ninety days due to stress, infections, bacteria, or inflammation. Why not just use X-rays instead? Well, X-rays can't see the depths of your gum pockets, only bone levels (for now—AI is coming!).

Gum measuring shows us if you have gum recession (exposed roots, which is also bad), healthy gums, or pocketing (disease). So, sorry, but it's for your own good. Second, it's a legal thing. Legally and clinically, your dentist has to diagnose what type of cleaning you're getting during your appointment, even if it's just a standard-normal-there-are-no-problems-here cleaning. Measuring your gums provides that diagnosis. So don't blame us. That's something else to blame on the government.

And if it hurts and you bleed, then blame yourself.

Honest, it's not normal for gums to bleed, ever. I've lost track of how many patients say their gums never bleed when they floss. I'm sure they're telling the truth. And the reasons why they don't bleed are either (a) they're not flossing or (b) they're not flossing correctly. If gums are infected, when floss gets to the base of the gum pocket, that will trigger blood. Most of the time, patients only go one to two millimeters below their gumline when flossing. If you have a five-millimeter pocket, you're not getting to the base of the pocket when flossing, which is where the bacteria (and blood) lie. You bleed when your dentist probes because they're getting down to the base of the pocket where the infection is. You don't. (You're welcome!)

Bleeding gums are never normal or okay. Every time a patient tells me they're bleeding because I poked at them with a sharp pointy thing, I take that same damn sharp pointy thing and poke their arm. Guess what? They never bleed.

Okay. I'm done with that rant (for a while).

Back to gum disease (which bleeding gums are a sign of— and *now* I'm done with my rant): if you have any form of it, waiting six months between exams and cleanings is much too long. Irreversible disease can set in during that time period and damage not just your gums but distant organs. So yes, you need to be probed at every visit. Also, if you're one who has a history of bleeding gums or periodontal disease, consider getting your cleanings every three to four months. And no, most of the time insurance won't cover those visits. But it doesn't mean you do not need them!

BREATHING MATTERS

Your dentist should be aware of how breathing affects your oral health and will want to examine your airway. Frankly, when you're in their chair is the perfect time to do it, as the dentist or hygienist has a clear view of the anatomy of your airway. They can easily identify if you are at high risk of having an airway health issue and provide a Mallampati score (see Chapter 12).

Other signs they'll look for are crowded teeth due to small jaws, broken teeth from grinding at night, and severe erosion from acid reflux. These are all signs of an airway problem. Sometimes your dentist can help with whatever the problem might be, like by supplying you with a mandibular advancement device. But something important to remember here is that your dentist doesn't need to be, and probably isn't, an expert in things like acid reflux or how mouth breathing can affect you. They are not looking at these issues to diagnose you with anything; they're just looking to see if something's wrong within their domain (your mouth) so that you can get the help you need from the right professional.

TESTS ON REPEAT

Your dentist may want to repeat tests for bacteria that you've had done before. One of the crappy things about bacterial infections is that you don't become immune to them. If you tested positive for Fn and were successfully treated for it or otherwise healed from it, that doesn't mean you won't get it again. In fact, research from the people over at OralDNA has discovered that bacteria typically repopulate within twelve months. Especially so if someone in your family is not as diligent with their oral care as you are. Swapping spit with them will reinfect you almost immediately.

Yeah, it's disgusting. But at least now you know, and you know what to do: never kiss anyone again. Just kidding; you need to let your dentist repeat the test! They might catch it early enough that they can eliminate it before symptoms show in your gums (or somewhere else in your body).

MAINSTREAM THE C-WORD

Your dentist should also do an oral-cancer screening—with the proper technology, not just a peek down the gullet—ideally every six months. And when they do, ask for the HPV saliva test that OralDNA Labs offers; this information is crucial for the early detection of oral cancer!

GET (RE)SCHOOLED

Like I said, we know you're not telling the truth when you say you brush twice a day and floss every day (it doesn't take a DDS to tell that if your gums are red, swollen, and bleeding). Usually, we're too polite to call you out on your bull; instead, we'll pretend like we believe you and just "review" how to properly brush and floss your teeth.

I often think it's funny when someone says, "my gums never bleed at home." It's even funnier when they complain about something not getting any better since their last visit. I'll remind them gently that they only see me 2 to 4 days out of 365, and they're responsible for the other 361 to 363! No one expects to win a bodybuilding competition when they only work out two days a year. So I don't know why anyone would think they'd have beautiful pearly whites and healthy gums by only going to the dentist twice a year.

You also shouldn't be expecting those beautiful pearly whites and healthy gums if you're eating a crappy diet. So it's possible your dentist or hygienist may want to provide a little nutrition and supplementation counseling too. Look, we dentists don't know everything about all medical possibilities. After all, if we graduated from university, we didn't continue on for more and more degrees. However, we know mouths. We can recognize when something's gone awry or if we have suspicions about what could be happening elsewhere in your body because of what we find in your mouth.

Take advantage of what we do know. And if we refer you to go to another doctor, GO!

DON'T BREAK UP WITH YOUR PCP

I hope you realize by now that it's not a matter of hubris when I say your dentist can save your life. But that doesn't mean you can skip seeing your primary care doctor at least once a year. And it certainly doesn't mean your dentist can be a substitute for any other specialist. Go to those other professionals when you need to. And if you don't have any in your contacts, ask your dentist. We have a network of clinicians we can lean on to help support your oral-systemic health. We'd be happy to connect you with them.

Meanwhile, think of what your dentist can do with all the tools and tests I've mentioned in this book as a form of early intervention. Things in the mouth don't cure themselves. If your dentist sees something that's a little off, they'll do what they can to help. But they can only treat what's in the mouth; if whatever is there could be causing a problem elsewhere, you need to go to a different doctor for that care.

Don't take a wait-and-see approach to whatever your dentist might find. Keep in mind that old phrase, *an ounce of prevention is worth a pound of cure.* Don't be tempted to wait and see if whatever's showing up under a VELscope is cancerous; have it checked out! Don't brush off high blood pressure at the dentist's office being a result of you being nervous to be there. Get checked out!

A wait-and-see approach will lead to more costly treatment down the road, not to mention more time and energy drained from you (and more stress!). And if you have any kind of condition like diabetes where you should see your specialist more frequently than once a year, then by all means do so.

I also recommend patients find PCPs who value oral health and will recommend the patient find and see a dentist when they are diagnosed with a comorbidity. It is critical that you have a complete team of providers to help keep you well. If your PCP has never recommended a dental checkup, I would encourage you to ask their opinion on the value of oral health.

But that doesn't mean the patient is off the hook. You have your own set of responsibilities to attend to, remember. So let's end the book by making your Personal Wellness Plan.

I hope I've inspired you to take that action and make a commitment to improving your oral health so you can improve your overall health and well-being. To help you make that commitment, consider signing this one here and/or visiting katieleedds.com to download your Personal Wellness Plan and for more resources:

I commit to doing the following by this date _____:

1. Find Dr. Right Dentist.

    My advice is to interview three dentists before deciding on Dr.
    Right. Look up functional or bio dentists as they are well versed
    in the oral microbiome

2. Pre-schedule at least two exams over the next year.

    We all get busy; I know! And the dental office gets busy—their
    office schedules will get booked up, making it difficult for a last-
    minute cleaning appointment.

    I recommend at least three cleanings a year if your gums are
    healthy, and four if you have gum disease.

    Regardless, you should schedule two exams each year.

3. Schedule my annual physical with my PCP to include com-
    plete blood work.

    Screen for ApoE4.

4. Take a home sleep test to rule out OSA. If negative, I will
    purchase mouth tape.

5. Purchase (check when complete)

    _____ Electric toothbrush

    _____ Water pick

_____ String floss

_____ Gentle mouthwash

_____ Mouth tape (if you do not have apnea)

_____ Tongue scraper

I commit to doing the following every day:

1. Brush morning and night for two minutes. (Set brush to deep clean or gum therapy if you have gum disease.)

2. Floss at minimum nightly. (I'll place the floss where I'll see it to easily remember.)

3. Engage in a stress-reduction technique. I will choose (circle as many as desired).

   Meditation or breath exercises (download an app, if necessary)

   Journaling

   Create a gratitude practice

   Thirty minutes of daily exercise

4. I will create a sleep routine where I

   stop caffeine at _____ o'clock

Shut off all glowing screens and turn the phone on do-not-disturb (or place it out of my bedroom) by _____ o'clock.

Be in bed, with lights out at _____.

Other activity to encourage my body to relax: _____

Supplement with melatonin and/or magnesium.

I commit to getting more movement by

1. Walking for _____ minutes each week.

2. Running for _____ minutes each week.

3. Biking for _____ minutes each week.

4. Weight training to increase my metabolism and decrease my risk of osteoporosis for _____ minutes each week.

5. Doing yoga for _____ minutes each week.

6. Doing Pilates for _____ minutes each week.

I commit to amending my diet by

1. Eliminating two "bad" things from my diet.

   I will no longer eat or drink _____.
   I will replace it with _____.

I will no longer eat or drink _____.

I will replace it with _____.

2. I will ensure I get enough fiber every day through this source: _____.

3. I will eat as many vegetables as I can stomach.

4. I will add this healthy fat to my diet: _____.

5. I will supplement with (circle all that apply)

Vitamin A.

Vitamin D_3 with K_2.

Vitamin C.

Curcurmin.

Fish oil.

Prebiotics.

Probiotics.

Magnesium.

Conclusion

THERE YOU HAVE IT! EVERYTHING YOU NEED TO KNOW to better your health, live longer, and keep money in your pocket. And it's so simple, right? Just a few minor/basic changes can make exponential improvements in your oral health and overall wellness.

If you've made it this far, your head is filled with stories about how people were able to turn their lives around and find optimum health by focusing on their oral health. You understand why inflammation is the root of all evil and how your poor oral health often has a causative role in many diseases, a supporting role in others, and a consequence for others.

Hopefully, you've made an appointment with your dentist to see what other ways they can help you improve your oral health and save you bucks in the long term. Think about this: for every dollar invested in preventive dental care, it's estimated that people can save between eight dollars and fifty dollars in future treatments.[87] That's a fifty times return on investment! Not even the market can do that!

---

87   University of Illinois Chicago College of Dentistry, "The Value of Preventative Oral Health Care," November 2, 2016, https://dentistry.uic.edu/news-stories/the-value-of-preventive-oral-health-care/.

My teenage accident wasn't just a one-and-done event. I still deal with the ramifications of that period of my life. I mean, I had my jaw wired shut for two months. I couldn't open my mouth for four years. Since then, I've had to get previous dental work fixed (it was done to the best ability of that time but needed rework). I've had teeth fail and get replaced with implants. I've had work done to ensure my airway health (my jaw was pushed backward in the accident, so my airway is pinched). And on top of all that, I battle with my IL-6 gene.

Although horrific, all of this has led me deeper and deeper into the field of oral health and wellness. I learned early on how quickly the body can turn to disease and shut down when it isn't being fed the proper foods and nutrients, how chewing our food properly affects digestion, and how important our teeth are for our smiles, self-confidence, and well-being.

I am making subtle, achievable adjustments to my daily life so that I can continue to serve patients for decades to come. Do not try to change everything all at once—small steps will have a massive impact! There are still many areas I can improve upon, but the goal is not perfection; it's progress.

It is my hope that you do follow through on the commitments you made in the previous chapter. And if you're looking for more inspiration or to stay up to date on the latest news in the oral health world, check out my website for information, blogs, and resources: katieleedds.com. You can also follow me on Instagram: @katieleedds.

About the Author

DR. KATIE LEE is a dentist, educator, mentor, and coach. A graduate from the University of Illinois at Chicago in 2010, Dr. Lee is a key opinion leader for Nobel Biocare and Ivoclar, is an international speaker, and has won numerous awards, including Top 40 under 40 dentists in America and receiving the Woman of the Year award at the Oral Systemic Medicine Conference in Germany. She has also been featured on local NBC and Fox News stations discussing her unique practice of incorporating technologies to treat oral-systemic health issues.

Dr. Lee has two passions in her profession: dentistry itself and making other dentists successful. For both, she underscores the need to focus on the oral-systemic health of patients. Her appreciation for the oral-systemic link comes from personal experience. An ATV accident as a teenager left her without many teeth and rendered her jaw immobile. Her recovery from that incident means she personally experienced how oral health affects systemic health. That life-altering dental trauma led her to specialize her dental practice around the mouth-body connection and dental implants. She focuses on improving periodontal health by using salivary diagnostics, improving sleep health, and restoring jaw function through the utilization of CAD/CAM and implant dentistry.

Dr. Lee lives in Aurora, Colorado. When not working or mentoring other dentists, she loves to be in the Rocky Mountains with her husband, Dr. Doug Lee, and two pugs, Ricky and Jules. She and her husband enjoy snow skiing, mountain biking, hiking, and scuba diving. She also has a passion for traveling and learning about new cultures.

To connect with Katie and see where she will be speaking next, visit her website: katieleedds.com.

Acknowledgments

WRITING THIS BOOK HAS BEEN SUCH A JOYOUS AND enlightening experience due to the amazing people in my life who have encouraged and challenged me throughout the years. I am passionate about this topic as a result of my own experience and feel incredibly blessed that I am able to share my knowledge with the world. My hope is to arm the public with knowledge that may not be mainstream so that they can take control of and improve their wellness and life span. Health and wellness are available to all.

The following people have contributed to this book in some way, and I want to sincerely thank them.

My husband, Dr. Douglas Lee. Thank you for standing by my side whilst building my dental empire across several states and constantly seeking and searching for new and innovative ways to improve my own wellness and that of my patients. Thank you for being there when things are good and when things are tough, always supporting me, and providing unconditional acceptance and security so that I can continue to get back out there and continue the grind of accomplishing great things. Thank you for allowing me to have big dreams and for providing a safety net for when I fall. Most of all, thank you for making life so incredibly fun.

Dr. Nicholas Burns. Thank you for modeling for me what being a dentist is all about. You served my life in two ways: you fixed my wreck of a mouth after my accident and also gave me a job in your office when I told you I wanted to be a dentist. I know you did not need extra help, but you did it to support my dream, and I am forever grateful. You showed me what it took to be an upstanding member of the community, how to care for patients, how to run a business, and how to motivate and lead a team. I credit my fast ramp as a dentist and a businesswoman to your early leadership.

Dr. Mark Erickson. Thank you for fixing my fuck face. I came to you mangled, and you disassembled the pieces and put me back together. My case was beyond complicated, and not something that could be fixed overnight, but you remained steadfast in your commitment to fixing me over four years despite your own health challenges. You always treated me with kindness and tenderness and showed me what it is to be an empathetic clinician and to put your patients first.

PDS / Steve Thorne. Thank you for being such a visionary and pioneer in the field of dental medicine. PDS remains at the forefront of oral healthcare, and Steve, your vision for medical-dental integration is far in front of both the medical and dental communities combined. Thank you for taking the chance on me when I graduated dental school as a twenty-six-year-old new grad and for the exposure you gave me to proven technologies that improve patient care.

My inaugural team, especially Dr. Kaz Talepbour, Kassy Wein, RDH, and Jasmine Mier, RDH. You all were instrumental in incorporating my practice modalities into daily practice with patients. Thank you for trusting my clinical expertise and for implementing it in the clinic daily. I created the vision, and you all helped bring it to life, helping thousands of patients improve their wellness.

Wendi Hill. Thank you for being my mentor in business and in life. You helped me rise above the weeds, see the bigger picture, and envision ways to expand my reach to help patients across the globe. You helped me see myself for what I am, a healer and a mentor to other clinicians, and I am forever grateful.

My EO forum. Thank you for challenging me in uncomfortable ways to grow and expand on my own. You helped me realize that I have infinite potential when I invest in myself. Thank you for widening my aperture beyond my dental world to see limitless possibilities to affect patients around the world. Thank you to Travis Luther for inspiring me to write a book and engage in possibility thinking, and for introducing me to Scribe.

Scribe Media, Lisa Shiroff. Thank you for organizing all of my passionate theories and practices into tangible and organized rhetoric for people to understand! This process was entirely enjoyable and simple because of your patience, hard work, and openness. The data changes daily, and I felt like I had a true partner in this process who was as dedicated to the mission and outcome as I was.